ART THERAPY WITH CHRONIC PHYSICALLY ILL ADOLESCENTS

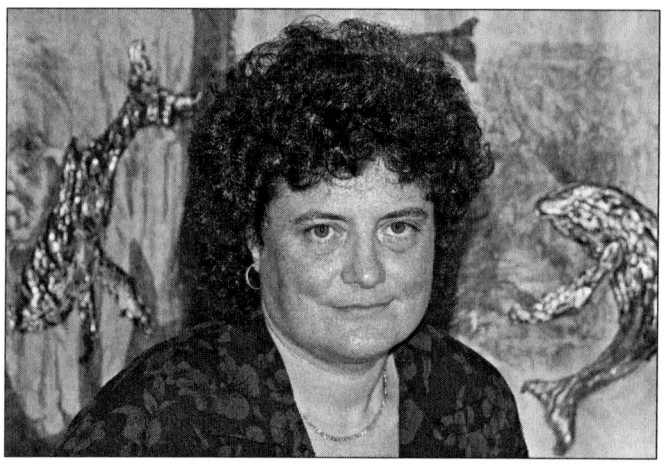

ABOUT THE AUTHOR

Ruth R. Luginbuehl-Oelhafen holds a medical degree from the University of Basel, Switzerland. She specialized in Pediatrics with a main interest in Developmental Pediatrics. She is a trained art therapist with a diploma from the Toronto Art Therapy Institute, where she was the recipient of the Martin Fischer Award for the best thesis. She introduced and taught the course for medical art therapy at the Toronto Art Therapy Institute. With her medical background in pediatrics, her clinical practice in art therapy has been heavily focused on the psychological impact of physical illness in children and adolescents. She is currently working in private practice in close collaboration with the department of pediatric palliative and bereavement care in a major children's hospital. As an active artist, she feels privileged to experience the healing power of her creative voice on a daily basis. In her work she focuses on the multiple facets and complexity of life.

ART THERAPY WITH CHRONIC PHYSICALLY ILL ADOLESCENTS

Exploring the Effectiveness of Medical Art Therapy
as a Complementary Treatment

By

RUTH R. LUGINBUEHL-OELHAFEN, M.D., DTATI

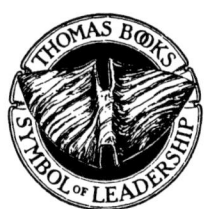

CHARLES C THOMAS • PUBLISHER, LTD.
Springfield • Illinois • U.S.A.

Published and Distributed Throughout the World by

CHARLES C THOMAS • PUBLISHER, LTD.
2600 South First Street
Springfield, Illinois 62704

This book is protected by copyright. No part of it may be reproduced in any manner without written permission from the publisher. All rights reserved.

© 2009 by CHARLES C THOMAS • PUBLISHER, LTD.

ISBN 978-0-398-07857-7 (paper)

Library of Congress Catalog Card Number: 2008046598

With THOMAS BOOKS *careful attention is given to all details of manufacturing and design. It is the Publisher's desire to present books that are satisfactory as to their physical qualities and artistic possibilities and appropriate for their particular use.* THOMAS BOOKS *will be true to those laws of quality that assure a good name and good will.*

Printed in the United States of America
LAH-R-3

Library of Congress Cataloging-in-Publication Data

Luginbuehl-Oelhafen, Ruth R.
  Art therapy with chronic physically ill adolescents : exploring the effectiveness of medical art therapy as a complementary treatment / by Ruth R. Luginbuehl-Oelhafen.
    p. cm.
   Includes bibliograhpical references and index.
   ISBN 978-0-398-07857-7 (pbk.)
  1. Art therapy for youth. 2. Chronically ill children. I. Title.

RJ505.A7L84 2009
618.92'891656--dc22
                                                                2008046598

*I wish to dedicate this book to all my patients,
who took me with them on their difficult journey and
who introduced me to the depth of their emotional struggle
in accepting and integrating their illness into their lives.*

PREFACE

Improved therapeutic interventions in medicine during the last 25 years have increased the chances of survivability for children with a wide range of conditions, including those in the newborn intensive care unit. In industrialized countries today over 85 percent of children born with chronic conditions will survive until at least the age of 20 years (Blum, 1992). As noticed by Golombek et al. (1989), adolescence becomes more complex as our social system becomes more technological and industrial. This is particularly true for physically impaired adolescents. Therefore, as professionals providing services in the medical health care system, we must expect to be increasingly confronted by the difficulties faced by these adolescents.

As a pediatrician I have learned that in early childhood, where the child is in a dependent position due on the one hand to his developmental immaturity, and on the other hand to physical illness, it is important to support the caregiving system. The better my understanding of family dynamics, the more I have the parents as allies and the more I can empathize and obtain cooperation and compliance. This will, in turn, facilitate the patient's course of treatment and his prognosis for a relatively smooth development.

But when the child is older, he should be encouraged to participate in decision-making and treatment. Communication with adolescents, however, poses a particular challenge for the doctor or other caregiving professional. At this transitional stage of their lives – no longer children, not yet adults – adolescents are experiencing many internal and external changes which, even in physically healthy teenagers, are accompanied by emotional turmoil over such issues as body image and social acceptance. For the teenager with a physical illness, these struggles are even more pronounced (Neinstein, 1991 & Hofmann, 1997). To reach independence while a chronic physical condition forces the individual back into dependence is a very difficult endeavor. In this situation it appears almost hopeless to get in control of one's own life, being constantly pushed back into the overwhelmingly controlling environment of the health care system. It seems impossible to leave the family core, when a chronic physical illness keeps the patient from socializing with peers.

Since I became a doctor I have tried various ways of reaching out to my adolescent patients. Too often, however, they choose not to communicate much and overtures about a recommended treatment or procedure evoke defiant reactions, a response typical of an age group that is striving for independence and suspicious of the expectations of anyone in a position of authority.

A communication vehicle that is potentially appropriate for this particular group is art therapy, due to its non-verbal approach (Linesch, 1988 & Riley, 1999). Art can represent a safe place in which to express and explore feelings. It may allow a person to present one's own reality when that reality is too emotionally charged to be expressed in words. Art offers an opportunity to become aware of and to observe one's own peculiar truth with more distance; it is as if the artist's product talks back to the artist. This is a kind of dialogue that takes place parallel to, and somewhat independently of, the relationship with the art therapist (Edwards, 1987).

As a pediatrician I am increasingly confronted with chronic physical illness in adolescence and its impact on the adolescent's future life. With my background in art therapy I am wondering whether this therapeutic approach can be helpful to this population in expressing and exploring its issues. During my search I found a great deal of literature about so-called medical art therapy with children and adults, but only a few case reports about adolescents. So I decided to focus more on this specific age group. For this work I have chosen a "client-centered" therapy approach, offering the client a non-threatening and non-judgmental environment rarely using directives. This therapeutic process is paced by the client and his actual needs, and therefore, gives him as much freedom and control as possible (Wadeson, 1980).

As a theoretical foundation for the case studies I used Erik Erikson's theory of Psychosocial Ego Development, since according to him development and maturation are based on resolving life crisis (Berzoff, 1996). I further consulted Neinstein (1991) and Hofmann (1997) concerning the issues of chronic physical illness in adolescence. Finally I included Wadeson's approach (1980) to art therapy in general, Linesch's (1988) and Riley's (1999) approach to art therapy specifically with adolescents, and Malchiodi's approach (1999) to medical art therapy.

The purpose of this book is to explore the effectiveness of art therapy as a primary intervention with an adolescent population with chronic physical illness – in this particular case, with adolescents in chronic renal failure either on hemodialysis, peritoneal dialysis or after kidney transplantation. The hypothesis is that art therapy (1) facilitates expression of emotions through artwork, ideally including verbal expression; (2) enhances self-esteem and identity; (3) helps them cope with their chronic physical illness; and (4) finally, offers an opportunity to vent anger and frustration (catharsis). By obtaining a safe place to explore issues related not only to the developmental stage but also to the conditions of chronic physical illness, these teenagers may begin to discover their individual strengths through art therapy, rather than dwell primarily on their individual weaknesses. In other words, the book will explore whether art therapy can be a means by which this population could be helped to accept and integrate their chronic physical conditions into their lives and to find an appropriate place in our society. In addition, this book will investigate whether art therapy could become a sanctuary, one in which the patient is allowed to keep control, to make his own decisions and to explore and develop a sense of freedom in an overwhelming controlling environment.

This book consists of four chapters with Chapter 1 providing an in-depth perspective on literature review and adolescence as a developmental stage. The psychological impact of chronic physical illness in adolescence, creativity and art therapy, medical art therapy, and the creative process is discussed. Chapter 2 studies methodology, independent variables, settings, procedures, materials used, and the gathering of data. Chapter 3 addresses case histories, their artwork, the short-term treatment group, and the long-term treatment group. Seven clients and examples of their artwork are presented. Chapter 4 discusses results, conclusions, and ideas for further studies.

R.R.L-O.

CONTENTS

Page

Preface vii

Chapter 1: Literature Review 3
    A. Adolescence as Developmental Stage 3
    B. The Psychological Impact of a Chronic Physical Illness in Adolescence 11
    C. Creativity, Creative Process and Art Therapy 22
    D. Art Therapy with Adolescents and Medical Art Therapy 27

Chapter 2: Methodology 39

Chapter 3: Case Histories and Artwork 51
    A. Short-Term Treatment Group 51
        1. Emma, female, 13 years 51
        2. Joan, female, 17 years 57
        3. Martin, male, 15 years 66
    B. Long-Term Treatment Group 73
        4. Abdul, male, 16 years 73
        5. Jayson, male, 13 years 98
        6. Katja, female, 12 years 124
        7. Nadja, female 13 years of age 148

Chapter 4: Discussion 177

Bibliography 201

Index 203

ILLUSTRATIONS

		Page
Figure 3.1.	*Wild Animals*, collage by Emma, 13 years.	54
Figure 3.2.	*Bud of a Flower*, clay sculpture by Emma, 13 years	56
Figure 3.3.	*My Family*, drawing by Joan, 17 years	61
Figure 3.4.	*Me and Andrew*, clay sculpture by Joan, 17 years.	61
Figure 3.5.	*My House and My Church*, drawing by Joan, 17 years.	62
Figure 3.6.	Untitled, mobile by Joan, 17 years	64
Figure 3.7.	*My Tree*, drawing by Martin, 15 years	70
Figure 3.8.	*A Bridge*, drawing by Martin, 15 years	71
Figure 3.9.	Untitled, watercolor by Abdul, 16 years.	77
Figure 3.10.	Untitled, watercolor by Abdul, 16 years.	81
Figure 3.11.	Untitled, charcoal by Abdul, 16 years	82
Figure 3.12.	Untitled, pencil drawing by Abdul, 16 years	84
Figure 3.13.	Untitled, pencil drawing by Abdul, 16 years	85
Figure 3.14.	*My Tree*, pencil drawing by Abdul, 16 years	88
Figure 3.15.	*Bridge Drawing*, pencil drawing by Abdul, 16 years	90
Figure 3.16.	*Da Vinci's Anatomical Wheel*, pencil drawing by Abdul, 16 years.	91
Figure 3.17.	*My Landscape*, pencil drawing by Abdul, 16 years	92
Figure 3.18.	*My Landscape*, continuation of pencil drawing by Abdul, 16 years.	93
Figure 3.19.	*My Landscape*, continuation of pencil drawing by Abdul, 16 years.	94
Figure 3.20.	*My Totem Pole*, pencil drawing by Abdul, 16 years	96

Figure 3.21.	*My Flags*, pencil crayon drawing by Jayson, 13 years.	103
Figure 3.22.	*The Rainbow*, watercolor by Jayson, 13 years	105
Figure 3.23.	*Fast Flying Balls*, watercolor by Jayson, 13 years.	107
Figure 3.24.	*Animals*, collage by Jayson, 13 years	108
Figure 3.25.	*Sports*, detail of the collage by Jayson, 13 years.	110
Figure 3.26.	*Sports II*, detail of the collage by Jayson, 13 years.	111
Figure 3.27.	*Cars*, collage by Jayson, 13 years.	113
Figure 3.28.	*In Honor of Hockey*, clay sculpture by Jayson, 13 years.	114
Figure 3.29.	Untitled, watercolor by Jayson, 13 years.	115
Figure 3.30.	Untitled, clay sculpture by Jayson, 13 years	117
Figure 3.31.	*My Tree*, watercolor by Jayson, 13 years	118
Figure 3.32.	*Michael Jackson's Glove*, papier maché sculpture by Jayson, 13 years	120
Figure 3.33.	*Happy Pumpkins*, clay sculpture by Katja, 12 years.	128
Figure 3.34.	*Bee Family*, clay sculpture by Katja, 12 years	129
Figure 3.35.	*Bird*, pipe cleaner object by Katja, 12 years	131
Figure 3.36.	*Teddy Bear*, clay sculpture by Katja, 12 years	132
Figure 3.37.	*Bird's Cage*, popsicle sticks object by Katja, 12 years.	133
Figure 3.38.	*Christmas Tree*, collage by Katja, 12 years	135
Figure 3.39.	*Snowman*, clay sculpture by Katja, 12 years	136
Figure 3.40.	*A Sitting Girl*, oil pastels by Katja, 12 years	138
Figure 3.41.	*Lucky*, oil pastels by Katja, 12 years	140
Figure 3.42.	Untitled, collage by Katja, 12 years	142
Figure 3.43.	Bowl, papier maché object by Katja, 12 years	143
Figure 3.44.	*My Personal Dream Catcher*, by Katja, 12 years.	145
Figure 3.45.	*Running Dog with her Puppy*, pencil drawing by Katja, 12 years.	147
Figure 3.46.	Untitled, mixed media collage by Nadja, 13 years.	153
Figure 3.47.	*My Mug*, clay mug by Nadja, 13 years.	154
Figure 3.48.	Untitled, oil pastels by Nadja, 13 years.	156

Figure 3.49. *Molly and Paul Holding Hands*, chalk pastels by Nadja, 13 years 157
Figure 3.50. Untitled, watercolor by Nadja, 13 years 159
Figure 3.51. *Styles of Ways of Clothing, Styles of Hair*, chalk pastels by Nadja, 13 years 160
Figure 3.52. *Under Sea*, chalk pastels by Nadja, 13 years 161
Figure 3.53. *Mr. Happy Potato Head*, papier maché container by Nadja, 13 years 167
Figure 3.54. *Mermaid*, therapeutic puppet by Nadja, 13 years. . . . 171
Figure 3.55. *My Dream Catcher*, Nadja, 13 years 174

PLATES

Plate 1. *A Landscape*, watercolor by Abdul, 16 years 45
Plate 2. *A Day of Celebration*, watercolors by Abdul, 16 years 45
Plate 3. *The Green Step Towards the Sun*, oil pastels by Abdul, 16 years 46
Plate 4. Untitled, chalk pastels by Abdul, 16 years 46
Plate 5. *Sports*, collage by Jayson, 13 years 47
Plate 6. *Sports II*, collage by Jayson, 13 years 47
Plate 7. *My White Rabbit*, oil pastels by Katja, 12 years 48
Plate 8. *Spring Flowers*, watercolors by Katja, 12 years. 48
Plate 9. Untitled, chalk pastels by Nadja, 13 years. 49
Plate 10. *Family Portrait*, chalk pastels by Nadja, 13 years. 49
Plate 11. *Mark's Story*, chalk pastels by Nadja, 13 years 50
Plate 12. *Our World, the Mermaids' World*, chalk pastels by Nadja, 13 years 50

ART THERAPY WITH CHRONIC PHYSICALLY ILL ADOLESCENTS

Chapter 1

LITERATURE REVIEW

A. ADOLESCENCE AS DEVELOPMENTAL STAGE

In talking about adolescence, the first thing to keep in mind is this: we are not talking about a homogeneous group, but rather a group that displays "wide variability in biological and emotional growth. Each adolescent responds to life's demands and opportunities in a unique and personal way" (Neinstein, 1991, p. 39). According to Neinstein, adolescence has been described as "a period of extreme instability" or "normal psychosis" (Neinstein, 1991, p. 39).

According to Anna Freud, "struggles of the ego to master the tensions and pressures arising from the Id lead in the normal case to character formation" (Freud, 1958, p. 257). She described "this battle between ego and Id as terminated by a first truce at the beginning of the latency period and breaking out once more with the first approach to puberty" (Freud, 1958, p. 257). "The individual recapitulates and expands in the second decennium of life the development he passed through during the first five years" (Freud, 1958, p. 256).

To further understand the developmental tasks of adolescence, I will use the theoretical framework of Erik Erikson's theory of Psycho-social Ego Development. I will have a look at his study of the developmental tasks starting from birth and leading to adolescence.

According to Erikson (1950/1963), the ego is shaped and transformed not only by biological and psychological forces, but by sociocultural forces as well. Erikson identified the ego strengths as well as the vulnerabilities that a person has to face during each stage of development. He stated that at each stage of psychosocial development there is the potential for the emergence of a unique kind of ego strength, as long as the individual faced and mastered the age-specific crisis with an age-specific concern at an age-specific time (Berzoff, 1996). It is important to understand that these stages are not sharply demarcated. They may overlap, regress, stagnate and catch up again, depending on an individual's life circumstances and his capability to cope. Childhood failures to master the age-appropriate developmental task limit the adolescent's ability to deal with the challenges of physical maturation, vocational search and self-definition. The result is a psychopathologic identity confusion in adolescence, which may even persist into adulthood (Jaffe, 1991).

According to Erikson, the first stage "Basic Trust vs. Basic Mistrust" (infancy, ages 0 to 18 months) – the oral stage according to Freud – is about establishing a basic trust between the child and the primary caregiver; therefore, the trust is to overcome "basic mistrust which is an inborn discomfort caused by the immaturity of homeostasis" (Erikson, 1950/1963, p. 247). The accomplishment of the "nuclear crisis leads to a general state of trust, which implies not only that one has learned to reply on the sameness and continuity of the outer provider, but also that one may trust oneself and the capability of one's own organs to cope with urges" (Erikson, 1950/1963, p. 248). "Consistency, continuity and sameness of experience provide a rudimentary sense of ego-identity" (Erikson, 1950/1963, p. 248) – of trustworthiness.

Erikson's second stage (early childhood, age 18 months to 3 years) – parallel to Freud's anal stage – is about "Autonomy vs. Shame and Doubt." Due to growing muscular maturation, this stage is one of ambivalence between "two sets of social modalities: holding on and letting go" (Erikson, 1950/1963, p. 251). Children at this stage need to achieve some sense of independence over their own body, including some sort of control over what is inside and outside of it. If a child comes to feel that his wish to have a choice and his urge for autonomy does not jeopardize his newly achieved "basic trust," he will gain some confidence and pride (Berzoff, 1996). At this stage the child's main struggles are control issues. He has to gain some sense of having the right to have control, but he also has to accept the fact that he will be controlled by outer forces as well. The child will have to confront first boundary issues. He will have to learn that within his social environment his freedom will end where his neighbor's (in this case his caregiver's) freedom begins. For the first time he will be confronted with differentiation between his and another's privacy (Erikson, 1968).

This stage, therefore, becomes decisive for the ratio of love and hate, cooperation and willfulness, freedom of self-expression and its suppression. From a sense of self-control without loss of self-esteem comes a lasting sense of good will and pride; from a sense of loss of self-control and of foreign overcontrol comes a lasting propensity of doubt and shame. (Erikson, 1950/1963, p. 254)

Erikson's third stage, "Initiative vs. Guilt" (play stage, ages 3 to 6 years), corresponds to Freud's Oedipal stage. The child enters a period rich in imagination and creativity, and begins to differentiate between concepts of the self and others. He faces the task of how to identify with his parents' and their society's values. The child now starts to develop an "'inner voice' of self-observation, self-guidance and self-punishment" (Erikson, 1968, p. 119) – the conscience as the cornerstone of morality (Erikson, 1968). "Initiative adds to autonomy the quality of undertaking, planning and attacking a task for the sake of being active and on the move, where before self-will more often than not, inspired acts of defiance or protested independence" (Erikson, 1950/1963, p. 255). Whereas in earlier stages the struggle for auto-nomy had concentrated on keeping rivals out, initiative in this stage leads to anticipation and challenge of rivalry in order to reach a superior position. Competition adds to creativity for initiative (Erikson, 1968). If the child encounters too little appreciation or even opposition to his endeavor, he will develop feelings of guilt, and will react with withdrawal and loss of self-confidence.

The fourth stage, which is termed "latency" according to Freud (school ages, age 6 to 11 years), Erikson has described as the stage of "Industry vs. Inferiority." The child now moves beyond the family nucleus and dives into social life, developing cognitive skills, play skills and social skills, including the ability to express and integrate his own feelings (Berzoff, 1996). It is the time to go to school, to learn, to develop competence, new physical and mental capabilities and to promote self-confidence. Children now are eager to make things together, to share responsibility and, therefore, to develop team skills, including the acceptance of rules. Through interaction with his peers, the child evolves ways to maintain self-esteem, developing increased ability to tolerate frustration. If for any reason the child is deprived of participating in social life and/or of developing a sense of achievement, he will grow feelings of inferiority.

Adolescence (ages 11 to 19 years), according to Erikson, is the stage with the psychosocial task of "Identity vs. Role Confusion." Adolescence is "a psychosocial stage between childhood and adulthood, and between the morality learned by the child, and the ethics to be developed by the adult" (Erikson, 1950/1963, p. 263). It is the stage of inner turmoil and instability, of ambivalence and inconsistency. Like Anna Freud, Erikson postulated that "in their search for a new sense of continuity and sameness, adolescents have to refight many of the battles of earlier years . . . only now with a new addition of genital maturity" (Erikson, 1950/1963, p. 261). Adolescents now become "primarily concerned with what they appear to be in the eyes of others as compared with what they feel they are" (Erikson, 1950/1963, p. 261). Individuals at this stage are looking beyond their parents for a sense of self and are prone to follow idols, apparently losing temporarily their own ideals. They are in a stage of suspended morality, while they are formulating new personal ideologies based on values that differ from their parents (Berzoff, 1996).

Acknowledging Erikson's statement about the sociocultural influence on human psychological development, I think we also have to consider sociocultural and economic changes in modern times while working with today's adolescents. Therefore, I will explore a more recent study published by Golombek and colleagues (1989), a group of North American psychoanalysts. As our social system becomes more technological and industrial, the roles and tasks assigned to adults become more complex. These role expectations, in turn, require a longer education and training and intensified experimentation for adolescents in preparation for adulthood (Golombek et al., 1989).

While Blos was one of the first psychoanalysts to subdivide adolescence in five subphases ("Preadolescence, Early Adolescence, Adolescence Proper, Late Adolescence and Postadolescence" [Jaffe, 1991]), Golombek's work is based on a model with three subphases – "Early, Middle and Late Adolescence" – each with specific developmental challenges (Golombek et al., 1989), including two transitional stages, before and after adolescence respectively. The first transitional stage before adolescence, so-called "Pubescence," includes all changes associated with movement from childhood into adolescence, especially physical changes. "Youth," the second transitional stage after adolescence, encompasses the changes associated with the progression from adolescence into adulthood (Golombek & Kutcher, 1990).

During "Early Adolescence" (ages 12 to 14 years), the child is dealing again with the early challenges that are rooted in Erikson's stage of

"Trust vs. Mistrust." The stress of new physical and psychosocial changes associated with altered adult reactions and expectations makes the child at this stage vulnerable. Preoccupied with rapid body changes, his former body image seems to be disrupted, which could be a source of anxiety (Hofmann, 1997). He narcissistically focuses attention on his body, and attempts to integrate rapidly increasing height, the changing shape, growing physical competence, rising sexual feelings and a new sense of power into his body image (Hofmann, 1997). His sexuality turns into a genital sexuality with increased interest in sexual anatomy and physiology, often provoking anxieties and questions regarding normalcy of functioning (Neinstein, 1991). The teenager begins to withdraw his interest in the parents as primary caregivers in order to explore his own environment. His feelings of mistrust for adults who seem ungiving and alien, change quickly with feelings of need, deprivation and hunger for attention and care. The result is difficulty in relatedness. He appears to be less self-confident and uncertain about his own beliefs, values and ideals. The internal self seems to fall apart. The child is anxious and depressed (Golombek et al., 1989). His cognition is still dominated by concrete thoughts; the teenager is not yet able to perceive long-range implications of current decisions and acts (Hofmann, 1997).

During "Middle Adolescence" (ages 14 to 16 years), the teenager seems to reactivate earlier issues of Erikson's "Autonomy vs. Shame and Doubt" stage. He is involved in a "process of personality recrystallization," taking in new identifications and self-representations while discarding old ones (Golombek et al., 1989, p. 501). Having experienced the majority of its pubertal changes, the body image as part of the personality starts to crystallize as well. Thus the middle adolescent still has to explore his sexual role. Therefore, great interest is invested in the ideal male or female appearance to determine what attracts the opposite sex. There is still little concern about reciprocity, commitment, and mutual caring, which will develop during later adolescence (Hofmann, 1997). With an increasing self-confidence and self-esteem, he develops a higher ability to assume and explore a variety of roles. Adolescents at this stage tend to present some sort of "omnipotent, grandiose and arrogant characteristics" (Golombek et al., 1989, p. 501). They rapidly gain competence in abstract thinking, but tend to revert to concrete thoughts under stress (Hofmann, 1997).

Finally, during "Late Adolescence" (ages 16 to 18 years) the adolescent has to face again the challenges associated with Erikson's "Initiative vs. Guilt" stage. With an increased ability of introspection, he appears also more willing to attempt to influence his environment. Demonstrating the highest level of curiosity in his outer world, the level of anxiety and depression seems to increase again. "Although identity structure seems to have been reestablished for most, the late adolescent is inexperienced regarding his reconstructed personality" (Golombek et al., 1989, p. 502). This inexperience causes discomfort, as the teenager struggles to integrate sexual, vocational, religious and political identities. By then the adolescent has established abstract thought processes, and is now capable of perceiving and acting on long-range options (Hofmann, 1997). Finally, with the relative consolidation of his identity, he is ready for more intimacy, the stage of young adulthood ("Intimacy vs. Isolation" in Erikson's terms).

In his longitudinal study, Golombek found three routes of passage through adolescence: "Stable/Clear Route" (clear of personality disturbances at each subphase of adolescence, 35% of average population); "Fluctuating Route" (clear during one subphase but disturbed at another, 40% of average population); and "Stable/Disturbed Route" (personality disturbances at each subphase, 25% of average population) (Golombek et al., 1989, Golombek & Kutcher, 1990). The course taken by any particular individual is dependent on such factors as: his constitution and temperament; his environment, including the amount of stress with which he is confronted; his social support system, and so forth (Golombek & Kutcher, 1990). Whether or not the stress factors of chronic physical illness influences the route of passage through adolescence is still a debate in literature (Capelli et al., 1989, Silver et al., 1990, Suris et al., 1996).

While I used Erikson's theory of Psychosocial Ego Development as a developmental framework helping to understand adolescence as a developmental stage, my therapeutic interventions as an art therapist are guided by an Object Relations psychodynamically oriented framework. The focus of Object Relations theory is on the complex relationship of self and others. It explores "the process whereby people come to experience themselves as separate and independent from others, while at the same time needing profound attachment to others" (Melano Flanagan, 1996, p. 127). Object Relations theories focus on the interaction individuals have with other people, and how he/she internalizes these interactions. Therefore, it includes "the whole internal world of relations between self and other, and the way in which others have become part of the self" (Melano Flanagan, 1996, p. 128). The word "object" traditionally is used for person.

Winnicott (1956), a major Object Relations theorist, believed that for a healthy psychological development

> important needs have to be met including the need to be seen and valued as a unique individual, to be accepted as a whole with both good and bad aspects, to be held tight and to be let go, and to be cared for, protected, and loved. (Melano Flanagan, 1996, p. 130)

Like the body takes in food in order to grow by metabolizing protein, fat and carbohydrates, the psyche takes in experiences with other people and processes them to become part of the psychological self.

Winnicott (1956) was especially interested in the capability of being together as a prerequisite for the ability to be alone and enjoy separateness. He stressed the importance of inner representations of others by internalization of good objects as a condition for this kind of healthy independence. The inner world has to be peopled with enough comforting figures, in order to develop the capability to be alone, or even enjoy solitude. According to Winnicott (1956) only a "good enough mother" (or caregiver) can create a "holding environment" necessary for the internalization of experiences with good objects (Melano Flanagan, 1996). A "good enough mother" is capable "for attunement to the baby's changing developmental needs" (Melano Flanagan, 1996, p. 138), without being neither neglective nor overprotective. She is able to adapt and change according to the changing needs of her child, and the growing child's decreased dependence (St. Claire, 2000). She offers her baby a "holding environment" subtle enough to be protective without being overly limiting.

Winnicott (1956) created the term the "transitional object." He observed that children in their attempt to move towards a state of separateness often use well-defined objects or rituals to sooth themselves in absence of their "good enough mother." "These 'transitional objects' offer ways for the child to hold onto the internal representations of others when she is not yet able to do so on her own" (Melano Flanagan, 1996, p. 138). The "transitional object" is a bridge to the possible existence of a beloved person even in absence.

Winnicott (1956) further stressed the importance of flexibility and genuineness of attachment to nurture the "true self," the core of a personality. "The 'true self' is the repository of individuality, uniqueness, difference" (Melano Flanagan, 1996, p. 140).

The True Self cannot emerge if the child feels she must be exclusively attuned to the needs of others in the family system and if she needs to be a certain way in order to be recognized and acknowledged. Instead the child may develop a False Self, one that seeks to suppress individuality and molds itself to the needs of others. This False Self, trying so hard to be responsive and to take care of others, ultimately becomes overly compliant. (Melano Flanagan, 1996, p. 140)

In summary, Object Relations theorists focus on the individual's internal world, which comprises representations of self and others, representations formed by ideas, memories and experiences in interaction with the external world. As therapists we are objects of this external world. By trying to develop a working alliance with the client, we are building a new relationship with him/her.

An object relations-oriented approach to treatment is often particularly useful in understanding and treating an adolescent population. Although adolescents struggle with conflicts related to authority and dependence, they still have very strong need for control with a reliable object. The art therapist can provide the adolescent with a non-judgmental, non-critical and reliable adult who they can go to with their concerns and problems, which they may not be able to, or elect not to discuss with their parents. In this environment they can test out behavior, explore ideas, thoughts and feelings they may not be able to express elsewhere. Also they are provided with a holding environment, in which they can learn to understand aspects of themselves, their feelings and their relationships. They maybe provided with a new or different object experience.

For the chronic ill teens, such an experience is control. They often struggle with intense conflicts about their body, illness, self-esteem, and so forth, which they are not able to discuss or share with anyone else. The opportunity to connect with an adult in a new way is often very helpful. In art therapy these teens can use the relationship with the therapist, the artwork, and the experience to learn more about themselves, their illness, coping styles, and enhance their capacity for relatedness with others.

B. THE PSYCHOLOGICAL IMPACT OF A CHRONIC PHYSICAL ILLNESS IN ADOLESCENCE

Successful development occurs through a process of continuous focusing and engaging in relevant developmental tasks. For chronically ill adolescents, however, stressors and tasks occur simultaneously. These adolescents must strive to maintain a delicate balance between appropriate developmental progression and physical health (Seiffge-Krenke, 1998). In general, the existence of a major life crisis such as a chronic physical illness during adolescence is likely to exaggerate the challenges of this developmental stage (Eiser, 1993). This impact is not only dependent on the individual's variability in ego-strength, stability and developmental stage, but on such factors as age of onset, course, visibility and prognosis of the chronic illness. In addition one has to consider the individual's support system (family dynamics, school environment, sociocultural relationships, friends, etc.) (Neinstein, 1991).

One would expect a chronic physical illness to have the biggest psychological impact on the body image of an individual. However, research suggests that chronic physical disease per se does not seem to have a negative impact on body image (Neinstein, 1991; Hofmann, 1997). Rather, there seem to be many factors that determine the psychological impact of chronic physical illness:

1. *Age of onset of the disease*: In general, the younger the child when first affected, the less disruptive the disease will be in a developmental sense. Congenital conditions or those with early childhood onset usually are well-integrated into identity, achieving a satisfactory adaptation by the time the child reaches adolescence. But in later stages like adolescence, the problems increase significantly. "Adolescence, however, is a time of exceptionally active intrapsychic reorganization and the additional stress of chronic illness . . . can overwhelm integrative functions already working at maximum capacity" (Hofmann, 1997, p. 741). With the onset of a disease in early adolescence the teenager's biggest concerns often are about body image and sexual functioning. Delayed puberty and pubertal growth spurt, or bodily malformations can create increased anxieties over sexual functions and sexual relations. The lack of growing physical competence may cause segregation from peers, and therefore add to an inferior self-image. This can contribute to lowered self-esteem, increased absences from school and

other social activities. As a result, it causes the teenager in this stage to become angry and/or depressed. Therefore, the more visible the disease the bigger the psychological impact in this age group (Neinstein, 1991). For those who are struck by a physical illness in middle adolescence, all of the problems described above also hold true, but they can often be more extreme since middle adolescence is the most devastating time for a chronic illness to strike. An adolescent in this phase is involved with separation, peer interaction, and sexual attraction. The consequences of a chronic disease have a very disruptive effect on the adolescent's natural urges (Neinstein, 1991). "At the age when even the healthiest young person feels different from peers and feels 'no one understands me,' the teen with chronic physical illness often feels even more removed from the mainstream" (Blum, 1992, p. 365). In addition, his feelings of omnipotence and personal invulnerability – typical traits for middle adolescence – are hurt. That may cause the adolescent to be reluctant to accept the diagnosis of a life-long or potentially fatal disease. With this reluctance goes a denial of the consequences of the disease, and the refusal to comply with treatment (Eiser, 1993). For those who develop a chronic illness in late adolescence, they usually go through less turmoil. The teenager at this stage will have already gained some self-confidence and identity. Concerns are focused on vocational and educational plans, financial resources, prospects for living independently, sexual function and future sexual relations (Neinstein, 1991).

2. *Degree and type of impairment*: A seriously impairing condition seems to have the biggest impact in middle adolescence as this is the time of heavy investment in emancipation and independence (Hofmann, 1997).

3. *Degree of visibility of the disease*: Directly visible conditions may cause a sense of personal devaluation and diminished self-esteem, especially in early adolescence. As a result there is a tendency for self-protective withdrawal and social isolation, or provocative acting-out in defense against possible rejection (Hofmann, 1997).

4. *Prognosis of disease*: The stress of uncertainty has the bigger impact than that when the course of the disease is known, even when leading to death (Boice, 1998; Blum, 1992).

5. *Course of illness*: Diseases with a fluctuant course with remissions and relapses are a bigger burden compared with chronic persistent conditions (Boice, 1998; Blum, 1992).

6. *Family issues*: The response of the family is a significant factor in the adolescent's compliance and adaptation. The parents may have to cope with the following: (1) guilt at causing renal failure, (2) fatigue and burnout associated with constant care and appointments, (3) inadequacy at not being able to help or fix the problem, (4) frustration with the medical establishment for no cure, (5) overprotection versus being too lenient, (6) marital stress, (7) rivalry between the sick child and his siblings, and (8) behavioral issues of neglected siblings, and so forth. Frequent trips to the hospital, daily home dialysis (hemodialysis and peritoneal dialysis) interfere with family schedules, school and vacations (Taylor, 2000). The more parents are able to be supportive in a way that achieves an appropriate balance between the required management of the disease and the teen's developmental needs, the smoother the adolescent will adapt. Often it is difficult for parents to provide required support in management of disease, avoiding the risk of overprotectiveness. Financial concerns may make the situation more difficult (Hofmann, 1997).

One of the main developmental issues in adolescence is the individual's conflict around autonomy and dependence. According to Boice (1998), autonomy is part of psychological well-being. "Achievement of autonomy depends on many factors, including the willingness of family and friends to allow the individual to take chances and realize personal potential" (Boice, 1998, p. 933). Therefore, to fully understand the independence struggle of an adolescent with chronic physical illness, we have to distinguish between "disability" and "handicap." In Blum's (1992) words (p. 366), "A disability is a restriction in functional capability imposed by physiology; a handicap, on the other hand, is determined by the social context coupled with the functional capability." In other words, while the teenager has to accept, to learn to cope with, and to adapt to a disability, the environment can help the adolescent in dealing with a handicap. Therefore, autonomy is dependent on the affected teenager's adjustment to the disease on the one hand, and on his support system on the other hand.

It is important to differentiate between two categories of autonomous behavior in the context of chronic illness. The first concerns autonomous behavior in a general sense, relevant to all individuals and relating to everyday issues. The second concerns responsible behavior specific to the management of the disease (Eiser, 1993). With regard to the first category, the disabled teenager should not be treated differently than his healthy peers. However, we have to keep in mind that the chronic condition may have a negative impact on self-confidence as it relates to the achievement of life's daily tasks. The second category is a more complex issue and is very much dependant on the cognitive development of the patient, and the onset, kind, course and prognosis of the disease. The more the teenager is able to understand the disease and its consequences to their full extent, the more he may be ready to take over responsibility in the disease's management, and therefore, will show reliability in compliance. Both categories of autonomy have to be achieved in the developmental process of maturation, paced by the adolescent's individuality.

This quotation by Blum (1992, p. 367) is an appropriate summary of this paragraph:

> We talk about development during the teenage years as a movement from dependence *to* independence. In truth, it is a movement from dependence *through* independence *to* interdependence." I think that independence is not synonymous to autonomy. Rather, to function within the frame of this interdependence means to be autonomous.

At this point I would like to focus on the process of achieving autonomy in the management of a disease that strikes during adolescence. The teenager goes through a process of adjustment after disclosure of the diagnosis of a chronic illness that is very similar to what Kuebler-Ross describes as the transitions people go through when dealing with death. Those stages are "denial – isolation," "anger," "bargaining," "depression" and finally "acceptance" (Gabriels, 1988; Kuebler-Ross, 1969; Weldt, 2003). Hofmann describes five phases of adaptation: Phase 1 extends from the first few days after disclosure of the diagnosis through the first week. Initial disbelief and shock is characteristic. The adolescent in his helplessness, with his anxiety over having lost control, and his unconscious fears of possible devaluation and loss of esteem, reacts with denial, depression, regression, anger and social withdrawal. Phase 2 extends from approximately the second week through the first month. The adolescent's biggest concerns are about physical integrity, body image, sexual identity, independence, peer acceptance and self-esteem; in other words, issues typical for this age but now in the context of a more complex situation of illness. Regression, resistance towards taking responsibility, reluctance to re-engage with peers, and anger and frustration are common reactions. Phase 3 extends over the second and third month after onset. The teenager is mainly concerned about re-entering the mainstream of life, fearing devaluation and rejection. Behavior varies from avoidance of usual activities to testing the parameters of his altered lifestyle and compromised independence. Rebellion against the limitations of disease-management requirements and testing out through non-compliance and, therefore, through disease exacerbation are often observed reactions. Phase 4 extends through the first few years after onset. By this time the adolescent's perception of the disease should be relatively realistic. Still concerned about previously listed issues, now he begins to contemplate possible future effects of the disease, and to develop adaptive coping, including reintegration into normal activities. At this point the teenager is ready to take a more active part in the management of the disease. Phase 5 extends through late adolescence into young adulthood. The patient begins to focus on acquisition of an adult level of autonomy, career plans, interpersonal relationships, and so forth. In general, the better the earlier conflicts have been resolved, the better the patient will adapt to his disease.

However, it is very important to keep in mind that these phases rarely are linear and chronological phenomena. Patients tend to go back and forth, regress, move ahead or skip part of phases only to get back to them later. As therapist it is important to acknowledge caution in using these phase-oriented schemes in order to remain as flexibly attuned to the patient as possible, and to avoid misleading assumptions and expectations (Kuebler-Ross, 1969).

Lazarus and Folkman define coping as cognitive and behavioral abilities to respond to any kind of internal or external forces or stressors (Eiser, 1993). Two types of coping strategies are described: (1) "Problem-focused" or "Primary control" concerns the attempt to change or control some aspects of the stressor or the environment, (e.g., taking an active part during a painful treatment of a disease, and therefore, have more control), and (2) "Emotion-focused" or "Secondary control" concerns the attempt to manage or regulate the negative emotions associated with stressors (e.g., trying to control anxiety or fear through relaxation exercise done before the painful treatment) (Eiser, 1993). Both coping strategies are seen within the same individual, independently of the kind of stressor (disease-related or daily life-related stressors). Depending on factors like the individual's age and temperament, past experiences with coping styles and family traditions, one or the other style may be dominant. A change in children's use of coping strategies during development has been noticed. With increasing age and maturation, the emotion-focused coping becomes more dominant. However, the adolescent has first to become aware that emotions can be brought under personal control to a certain extent (Eiser, 1993).

Adolescents cope with their chronic physical illness by using a wide range of adaptive and maladaptive defense mechanisms. These defense mechanisms may be employed unconsciously, but the result is that negative emotions are made more controllable by placing them into manageable proportions. In other words, they help the patient move back toward homeostasis (Hofmann, 1997). The following defense mechanisms have been described in adolescents who have to deal with chronic physical illness:

1. **Intellectualization**: This behavior separates the realities from the disease from the emotional impact. While suppressing the emotional part, the factual aspect is dealt with rational objectivity, as if it had nothing to do with the patient.
2. **Compensation**: Lost qualities are substituted by new constructive activities.
3. **Displacement**: Concerns about oneself are substituted by concerns about something or somebody else.
4. **Projection**: Self-blame and guilt over a situation are unconsciously shifted onto someone or something else.
5. **Regression**: In order to avoid unbearable responsibilities, the patient moves back to a more child-like dependence.
6. **Denial**: Threatening aspects of the disease are suppressed, as if they did not exist. (Hofmann, 1997; Neinstein, 1991)

Behaviors such as acting out or panic attacks are often seen when uncontrollable fears and anxieties overwhelm the patient.

> The ultimate adaptive goal is insightful acceptance of the chronic conditions and its limitations, but this is rarely accomplished during the adolescent years and may take well on into adulthood to achieve, if ever. (Hofmann, 1997, p. 743)

To complete the list of psychological impacts of a physical illness I will explore the adolescent's behavior of secondary gain. Secondary gain describes the phenomenon that is often observed with chronic illness (physical and/or mental), where the patients receive benefits or satisfactions as a result of their disabling conditions. An adolescent with chronic illness can use his illness to avoid issues that frighten him (e.g., dependence, separation, sexuality, etc.); he may enjoy the absence from school; he may also develop a feeling of entitlement or right for special treatment; within a family dynamics he may exploit the situation by being spared from duties and responsibilities; and so on. Secondary gain from illness can be a very powerful phenomenon and it can be a major obstacle to adaptive or positive life changes. While the adolescent may have limited conscious awareness of the gain of the illness, the process often is largely unconscious. It is very important that clinicians consider the impact of secondary gain in the assessment and treatment of any individual with a chronic illness (Mackinnon & Michels, 1987).

At this point I would like to focus more specifically on my population, adolescents with the condition of chronic renal failure. To understand the psychological impact of this condition to its full extent, we need some medical background information.

Chronic renal failure (CRF) describes a condition in which the kidneys do not work properly anymore – that is, they do not perform the function of the elimination of toxic waste; the regulation of total body fluid balance, electrolytes (Sodium, Potassium) and minerals (Calcium, Phosphate); the regulation of blood pressure; the production of Erythropoietin (a substance important for the production of hemoglobin); the metabolism of vitamin D; and, therefore, the regulation of the bone metabolism, etc. The causes that lead to CRF are multiple (congenital dysplasia, acquired glomerulonephritis, vasculitis, interstitial nephritis, pyelonephritis, hereditary cystic kidneys, tumors, etc.), as our population showed. General clinical manifestation of CRF are edema, anemia/fatigue, anorexia/nausea, renal osteodystrophy/growth retardation, hypertension/headache, neuropathy with gross/fine motor delay, delayed sexual and cognitive development, menstrual irregularities/impotence, and skin problems (with itchiness due to the build-up of toxic wastes in the skin), as well as well-known drug side effects.

When talking about end-stage renal failure (ESRF) we are describing a condition in which conservative (non-invasive) treatment (remarkable dietary restrictions with limitation in fluid/salt intake, diuretic and antihypertensive medication, managing anemia and growth retardation) of CRF is not sufficient anymore. Renal replacement therapy like hemodialysis, peritoneal dialysis or kidney transplantation is necessary in addition to all above listed restrictions.

Each of the more invasive treatments has its specific advantages and disadvantages:

- **Hemodialysis**: This is a procedure, in which the blood circulates out of the body through a machine with a filter system and back into the body for about 3–4 hours, 3–4 times a week. The advantage of this treatment is that it brings a fast correction of fluid, electrolyte and metabolic abnormalities. It requires anticoagulation to prevent the clotting of the blood in the machine, special nursing skills and high surveillance during the procedure due to high complication rate (hypotension, dysrhythmia, muscle cramps, seizures). A vascular access has to be established, which requires sterile handling due to high risk for infections. In children, a central venous line with its tip in the right heart is surgically inserted, and needs careful dressing after each use. With these tubes attached to the chest the child has to follow certain restrictions in physical activities: no swimming, and no team sports with potential body contacts (hockey, football, soccer, etc.). Although physical activity is recommended, it has to be on a more individual basis (bicycling, jogging, etc.). Other big disadvantages are frequent trips to the hospital, frequent absence from school, impediments with regard to participation in social activities, interference with outings and holidays, which involves the whole family (Taylor, 2000).
- **Peritoneal Dialysis**: This is a procedure, in which a sterile solution (dialysate) is instilled into the peritoneal space. Waste particles are removed from the blood across the peritoneal membrane by diffusion during the 3–4 hours of dwelling of the fluid in the abdomen. Four to six times a day these dialysate bags have to be changed; that means the patient has extra fluid in his abdomen for almost the entire day, often causing discomfort with stomach pain and feelings of fullness. Although this relatively safe procedure is very time-consuming, it offers a certain independence from the hospital since it is usually done at home. As with hemodialysis, access to the body has to be installed surgically, and then handled in an absolutely sterile manner to prevent infections (peritonitis being the most fatal complication) (Taylor, 2000).

- **Transplantation**: This is a procedure, in which the patient will have an organ implanted, either from a living-related donor or a compatible donor who suddenly died (cadaveric). With increased scientific knowledge about immunosuppression, this kind of renal replacement therapy seems to be most successful. A careful, often very annoying assessment (including blood typing, HLA [human leukocytes antigen] tissue typing, antibody cross-match compatibility testing, beside all the diagnostic imaging, etc.) of the patient and the donor is required previous to surgery. In the case of a living donation, hospitalization and transplantation are carefully planned. In the case of a cadaveric donation, all the patient's test results will be added to an international waiting list. The patient must always be ready to reach the hospital within two hours of time. And he may have to wait for weeks or years, which makes the situation very stressful. Renal transplant surgery is the least complicated of the transplantation interventions and requires about 4–8 weeks of recovery in hospital. Immediately after surgery the immunosuppressive treatment has to be started. Since the risk for rejection is higher at the beginning, medical controls with bloodwork and biopsies are more frequent at the beginning, and looser later on. Associated problems with immunosuppression are high risk for infections, nephrotoxicity, neurotoxicity and (in longer terms) lymphoproliferative neoplasias (leukemia, lymphomas, etc.), beside specific drug side-effects for the particular drug used. Nowadays a transplanted kidney survives for about 10–15 years on average, and then has to be replaced by any kind of renal replacement therapy. That means that the younger the patient, the higher the risk for multiple transplantation (Kosmach, et al. 2000).

It is very important to understand ESRF as a chronic, life-threatening condition without real cure, since none of the above listed treatments offer a permanent rescue – a fact that has to be kept in mind when considering psychological impact.

During my literature search I could not find any studies on the psychological impact of ESRF in childhood and adolescence. I did, though, discover a few for adulthood. Although a lot of the age-related issues are quite different, some of them appear to be common to both young and old.

In their work with adult hemodialysis patients Buchanan and Abram (1984) describe mainly two stages of adaptation to the disease and its treatment. The initial stage includes an acute psychological response that is characterized by "hope for future well-being and anticipated benefits from increased efficiency" (Buchanan & Abram, 1984, p. 274). The concept of hemodialysis as a chronic lifelong treatment has not been established at this point of time. Gradually, however, this hope changes to fear of an unknown future. Withdrawal and reclusion from social contacts are common reactions. At this stage it is important to encourage the patient to ventilate his feelings. The chronic stage of adaptation is characterized by the realization that dialysis has become a way of life. Often "despair and doubt replace an overly optimistic expectation of the treatment" (Buchanan & Abram, 1984, p. 275). Regression and/or depression are common reactions.

During these stages of adaptation Buchanan & Abram (1984) noticed three main areas of conflicts:

1. *Independence*: While the patient has to accept the dialysis regimen and remains fully dependent upon a machine for the rest of his life, he is expected to assume the responsibilities of a healthy person in his "spare-time." "It is extremely difficult, however, to live a life with such duality of purpose. It is much more common to adopt one of the two extremes, either of which is considered by us maladaptive" (Buchanan & Abram, 1984, p. 277). On the one hand Buchanan and Abram are talking about an extreme dependent and submissive behavior, and on the other hand about an excessive independent and rebellious behavior.

2. *Identification with the illness*: Again, two extreme patterns of behavior are commonly seen. One extreme represents the "identifier" who becomes totally absorbed in hemodialysis and makes this treatment modality the purpose of his life; the other extreme is the "avoider" or "denier" who denies the severity or even the existence of his disease.

3. *Expectations*: Conflicts root in the difference between the patient's expectation of his life and the expectations of the medical staff. During both stages of adaptation the patient may "perceive the staff as constantly being at cross purposes to him," which can end up in mistrust (Buchanan & Abram, 1984, p. 278).

Stapleton (2000) categorized stressors connected with ESRF in physiological, psychological, role disturbance and life change. Physiological stressors are due to the toxic effect of uremia and include disturbances in body chemistry (altered body fluid and electrolyte homeostasis) and organ system disturbances (hypertension, anemia, osteodystrophy, etc.). Psychological stressors include body image, frustration in basic drives, fear of death and dependence – and independence conflicts. While sitting at the hemodialysis machine and watching the blood circulating, the patient comes to perceive himself as part of the machine – or to incorporate the machine upon which he is dependent for life into his body image (Stapleton, 2000). Sitting there "on the leash" conducting the blood from the body to the machine and back the dependence becomes almost literal. A body, which is intoxicating itself, not being able to clean the blood anymore, changes in value, which contributes to a disturbance in body image. Frustrations in basic drives like satisfaction of hunger and thirst, sexual drive and so on add to this problem. Role disturbances include the fact of being forced to eliminate social, family and occupational roles, leading to feelings of isolation and disengagement. Often, time for treatment interferes with other desirable life activities, and makes the planning for outings and holidays impossible. These and other lifestyle changes are even more pronounced for patients who wait for a cadaveric transplant and live in constant uncertainty and ambivalence (Stapleton, 2000). These stressors together with the characteristic symptoms of CRF (chronic fatigue, low energy level, nausea, itchiness, etc.) and the restrictions in diet and physical activity contribute to the feelings of powerlessness and helplessness. The disease process of CRF leading to ESRF itself is a factor over which the individual has little control. Even in kidney transplantation, the inability to control or predict the outcome of the transplant is a real cause of feelings of powerlessness. This occurs not only postoperatively, but also for the rest of the life, since the risk for rejection, although decreasing in time, is always real.

Clearly, ESRF treated with whatever modality has a huge psychological impact on an individual's personality and life. The way a patient is able to cope with these circumstances is very much dependent on his character, his social support system, his developmental stage and, last but not least, his own resources.

C. CREATIVITY, CREATIVE PROCESS AND ART THERAPY

Each individual needs to operate in a state of equilibrium. If this state is disrupted, the individual will first try to rely on coping mechanisms that have previously been successful. Adaptive or maladaptive, these familiar – and most often unconscious – inner resources are called upon in an attempt to lead the individual back toward homeostasis. But when usual coping patterns are inadequate, a crisis is identified, making new methods of responding necessary (Moos & Schaefer, 1984). The individual must then employ a more conscious ingenuity in order to find ways out of imbalance. And that is where creativity comes in to play. Creativity is described as a mental process that leads to solutions, ideas, artistic forms, theories and products that are unique. Creativity is not making art. Though not everyone is capable of becoming an artist, everyone is capable of being creative. "Throughout our lives we are engaged in an ongoing creative enterprise" (Wadeson, 1980, p. 4). "Creativity makes life worth living, gives life a meaning" (Winnicott, 1971). According to Malchiodi (1998) "Creativity is thought to include many or all of the following qualities: Spontaneity, playfulness, imagination, motivation, originality, self-expression, inventiveness, divergent thinking, and intuition" (p. 65). Creativity includes pushing limits, breaking down boundaries and rejecting accepted assumptions.

During a creative process the individual may start to recognize the limitations of his current ways of thinking. He may also start to question the ways in which he looks at the world. Humanistic Psychology emphasizes the importance of creativity, play and spontaneity in self-actualization. In other words, the creative process can help the individual to make life more meaningful, to enhance his ability to know himself, and to help him reach his potential (Malchiodi, 1998). "Creative people are known to be more independent, autonomous, self-sufficient, emotionally sensitive, assertive, self-accepting, resourceful, adventurous and risk-taking" (Malchiodi, 1998, p. 65).

There are strong connections between the creative process and the process of therapy, especially art therapy. Both are about solving problems, finding new solutions to old ways of feeling, thinking, interacting. Both provide opportunities of exploring and experimenting with new ideas. Both are acts of transformation and modification. And both involve an encounter with one's self. The creative process within a therapeutic setting leads to insight and self-awareness and, therefore, can be the beginning of personal change, growth and integration (Malchiodi, 1998). The process of art psychotherapy includes the client's and the therapist's creativity (Wadeson, 1980).

At this point I would like to focus on art therapy and how it works. There are two main definitions of art therapy. The first is based on the idea that art is a means of symbolic communication. This approach – often referred to as Art Psychotherapy – emphasizes the product itself as helpful in communicating issues, emotions and conflicts. In this kind of psychotherapy the art piece becomes significant in enhancing the verbal exchange between the client and the therapist (Naumburg, 1966). This approach is often associated with "insight-oriented therapy." By using open-ended questions the art therapist encourages the client to "free associate" about the art work. The goal is to address difficulties, and to help the client to deal with them (Wadeson, 1987). The art therapist therefore, needs to create a design of the therapy that serves the purpose, using appropriate directives, art materials, and so forth (Wadeson, 1987). A drawback to this therapeutic approach is that a certain level of functioning by the client is necessary in order for him to gain insight. This method is more often used with older children or adults.

The second approach to art therapy involves the belief that it is the creative process of art-making itself that has healing power. The term "Art as Therapy" refers to the idea that the process of making art is therapeutic (pioneer Edith Kramer, 1971, who was working mainly with children). In this context Wadeson (1980) uses the expression "client-centered therapy," in which the here and now is important, and the therapist's task is "to help to remove roadblocks to the natural flow of creativity" (Wadeson, 1987, p. 56). By providing a non-threatening and non-judgmental environment, the therapist's goal is to encourage the client to express himself at his own pace. The process of creating enhances pride, power and control, and finally self-esteem (Wadeson, 1987; Weldt, 2003). Since this therapeutic approach does not require capability for insight, it is more often used with children. In reality, most of today's art therapists integrate both approaches into their work in varying degrees (Malchiodi, 1998).

In 1966, Margaret Naumburg was one of the first pioneers to use art expression as a therapeutic modality. Following a psychodynamic approach, she postulated that "man's fundamental thoughts and feelings are derived from the unconscious and often reach expression in images rather than words" (Naumburg, 1966, p. 1) – a fact that Freud described in his dream work. The images that arise deal with unconscious conflicts, fantasies, fears and childhood memories, very much like dreams and daydreams. According to Naumburg, art therapy has a big advantage over verbal therapy because such symbolic images "more easily escape repression by what Freud called the mind's 'censor' than do verbal expressions" (p. 2). In other words, since our "unconscious speaks in images" (Naumburg, 1966, p. 2), any kind of verbal expression of unconscious material undergoes some sort of translation, a process which is perhaps more prone for censorship.

Naumburg (1966) added another advantage for art therapy: "When a forbidden impulse has found such form (as a picture) outside the patient's psyche, he gains a detachment from his conflict which often enables him to examine his problems with growing objectivity" (p. 3). Wadeson stresses the importance of the art product as a tangible object. According to her experience "it is often easier for resistant patient to relate to the picture (as an object) than to the self" (p. 10). She calls this process "objectification":

> Because feelings and ideas are at first externalized in an object. The art object allows the individual, while separating from the feelings, to recognize their existence. If all goes well, the feelings become owned and integrated as a part of the self. (p. 10)

Thus, this artistic product can be treated as a mirror of the client where he can discover his own self.

According to Wadeson (1980), during our development as human beings we think in images long before we have words. Therefore, much of our preverbal thinking is stored in images within ourselves. "That imagery probably plays a large part in early personality formation, the core experiences which influences subsequent layers of personality development" (Wadeson, 1980, p. 8). Bowlby's Attachment theory has become a major focus in more recent neuroscience research. It is believed that successful attachment between child and caregiver is critical to optimal development for specific parts of the brain. Siegel (1999) and Schore (1994) believe that "interactions between child and caretaker are right-brain mediated because during infancy the right cortex is developing more quickly than the left" (Malchiodi, 2003, p. 20). Siegel observes that the right hemisphere requires emotional stimulation to develop properly, whereas the left hemisphere requires language if it is to grow. Therefore, he adds, the output of the right hemisphere is expressed in non-verbal ways, like pictures, whereas the left hemisphere uses more verbal expression. According to this idea, art therapy may be an important means in working with emotional problems that are rooted in a preverbal stage (Malchiodi, 2003).

Another explanation as to why art therapy may be helpful, especially in traumatized clients, can be found in the way in which memories are stored. "There are two types of memory: explicit memory is conscious and is composed of facts, concepts, and ideas and implicit memory is sensory and emotional and is related to the body's memories" (Malchiodi, 2003, p. 21). Current speculations are that traumatic memories are excluded from the explicit storage, and therefore are not directly reachable. Art therapy, which, it has been argued, may have more access to the implicit storage than verbal therapy, may help to bridge the implicit and explicit memories and, therefore, help the client to explore these memories in a more explicit (conscious) way (Malchiodi, 2003).

Wadeson (1980) thinks art therapy has several advantages over verbal therapy. For example: She points to the permanence of the art product as unique to this modality of therapy. "The picture or sculpture is not subject to the distortions of memory (as words often are). It remains the same and can be recalled intact months or years after its creation" (Wadeson, 1980, p. 10). Reviewing art pieces at a later stage of art therapy, she adds, contributes to the "sense of the ongoing development that occurs in the therapeutic process" (Wadeson, 1980, p. 10). She further stresses the art's "spatial matrix." Unlike verbalization, which is a linear communication, "art expression needs not to obey the rules of language – grammar, syntax, or logic. It is spatial in nature" (Wadeson, 1980, p. 11). There is no time frame. Art has the ability to communicate relationships using shapes, color and lines in space (e.g., it is easier to describe relationships within a family in a visual [spatial] way, than in a verbal [linear] way) (Wadeson, 1998).

As mentioned before, pictorial projections are a method of symbolic communication between client and therapist. However, the art therapist is not supposed to interpret the symbolism of this art expression. Rather, the therapist's role is to encourage the client to discover the meaning of his art product by means of free association (Naumburg,

1966). Wadeson (1980) even warns against using questions too suggestive for specific answers. Instead, she recommends using open-ended questions. Furthermore, she postulates that the artwork speaks to both – the client and the therapist, but in different ways. Therefore, "what I (as art therapist) read in it is an echo of my own life experience" (Wadeson, 1980, p. 38).

As with all other therapeutic modalities it is very important for the art therapist to develop self-awareness into the therapeutic relationship. That means the therapist should be aware of personal issues with respect to transference and countertransference. This includes social and cultural issues, as well as earlier personal life experiences. According to Wadeson (1980), transference is an important tool in art therapy, as it is in other dynamic therapeutic modalities. She describes the therapist's role in a therapeutic relationship this way: By providing a supportive and non-threatening atmosphere the therapist facilitates an accepting, non-judgmental and understanding relationship. The therapy becomes a safe laboratory in which she encourages clients "to feel free to experiment, assuring them that here there are no prices to be paid for failures, that, in fact, failure can provide instructive learning" (Wadeson, 1980, p. 34).

Art therapy imposes some special factors in the therapeutic relationship. There is not only the relationship between two people, there is also the relationship with the art product. "As an expression of self it becomes an extension of the client and must be respected as such" (Wadeson, 1980, p. 38). Therefore, the art therapist has to be aware of the importance of how he regards, handles, stores and recalls the art work as an extension of his client. Furthermore, he has to be aware of countertransferential feelings towards the piece of art as well as towards the client.

Art therapy as a treatment modality is not based on one specific theoretical foundation. Art therapists tend to orient themselves to one of the main theoretical approaches (e.g., psychodynamic, humanistic, cognitive-behavioral, etc.) and to build their professional frameworks by borrowing ideas from one or several sub-orientations (e.g., Object Relations Approach, Self Psychology Approach, Jungian Approach, Psychosocial Approach, etc.) (Rubin, 1987).

Although still a young discipline, art therapy has found its way into mental health institutions, psychological services of schools, prisons, refugee centers, women shelters, hospitals, and so on. With increasing awareness of the importance of emotional well-being for the physical healing process, more and more hospitals offer this help not only for emotional disturbances but for physically ill patients as well (Malchiodi, 1998; Malchiodi, 1999; Malchiodi, 2003).

However, it is important to acknowledge the limitations and contraindications of art therapy. Limitations of art therapy with an adolescent population may be: (1) lack of interest in using visual art for expression; (2) high physical impairment, which makes it impossible to make art (e.g., tetraplegia, etc.); and (3) mainly in male clients lack of motivation due to a prejudice that art is only for females, children or "softies" (Moon, 1998).

There are a few contraindications demanding special caution in using art therapy. In patients with active psychosis or difficulties with reality testing, art therapy could be anxiety-provoking or encourage regression. Special caution is requested in using art therapy with patients suffering from severe post-traumatic stress disorder (PTSD), since depicting the trauma could re-enact the traumatic event (Merriam Beth, art therapist, personal communication, September 2001). In these cases art therapy may be most effective as an adjunctive treatment, in combination with medication and/or psychotherapy. Like any therapy or treatment it is essential that the therapist complete a comprehensive assessment to determine the best form of treatment. Of note is that at present time there is a lack of empirical literature on the efficacy of art therapy. Much of the support of art therapy is case-based and anecdotal evidence from clinicians.

Art therapy often is particularly useful for those clients who are resistant to or hard to reach through verbal therapy, or have difficulties putting things into words, and are open to visual art. Therefore, it usually fits well with children and adolescents (Wadeson, 1980; Malchiodi, 1998).

D. ART THERAPY WITH ADOLESCENTS AND MEDICAL ART THERAPY

In this chapter I would like to focus on art therapy as it relates to my study population: adolescents with a chronic physical illness. There are, however, only a few case reports that I could find in the literature about medical art therapy with adolescents – much more research has been done in medical art therapy with children and adults. As a result,

I have decided to split this chapter into three parts. The first will concentrate on art psychotherapy with adolescents. The second will focus on medical art therapy in childhood and adulthood. Finally, in the third section, I will give an overview of the few articles about medical art therapy with adolescents.

When talking about art psychotherapy with adolescents, it is important to remember that we are primarily discussing a population that exhibits behavioral and mental health issues, but usually is physically healthy. However, in my population these issues were not primarily the reason for the referral to art therapy. If behavioral issues were present, they were found to be in connection with their struggles with chronic physical illness.

According to Riley (2001), in general, regardless of the main issue, "the discrepancies between the adolescents' expectations, the expectations of the society, and the commercial image projected by the media is the source of much of the confusion of today's youth" (p. 55). That confusion makes it difficult for adults to establish relationships with the adolescents with whom they are working. In the therapeutic studio, teenagers can often be demanding, moody, destructive, self absorbed, provocative, disruptive, manipulative and inconsistent. They are unpredictable, seldom grateful and never satisfied (Moon, 1998). It is often "difficult to provide a non-confrontative, flexible form of therapy to the reluctant teenager who resists being in therapy" (Riley, 1999, p. 39). Riley (1999) states "imagery, as it is used in art therapy, is often the key of making an early alliance" (p. 39).

In general "teenagers are willing to draw and create art as freely as they resist talking to an adult" (Riley, 1999, p. 31). Indeed "drawing, or making marks, is in tune with adolescents' development . . . It is hard to restrain an adolescent's urge to 'make their marks.' Channeling this drive into productive communication can neutralize the battle over what to reveal or keep hidden" (Riley, 2001, pp. 55–56). Moon (1998) states that "art therapy with adolescents is a metaverbal treatment modality" (p. 21). He defines "metaverbal" as being "experiences that are beyond words" (p. 8), meaning that the "curative work of art therapy takes place in the interaction between the adolescent, the media, the image and the process" (p. 8). Riley (1999) also points out that language often is "a smoke screen behind which the adolescent can hide from adults. By inventing new words with specialized meanings, changing that vocabulary from month to month, the outsider is effectively excluded" (p. 57). However, this tactic can often be negated by turning to the visual communication that art therapy provides. Since adolescents are more prone to action than reflection, visual expression seems to be an appropriate tool of communication. According to Linesch (1988), "art expression as a developmentally appropriate modality, provides the adolescent with an ego-syntonic aid in his/her difficult struggle" (p. 7). However, as stated earlier, art therapy does not appeal to all adolescent individuals. Some teenagers may be particularly reluctant because art therapy may be experienced as infantilizing.

At this point I would like to focus on some of the features that are typical of art psychotherapy with adolescents – in other words, additional characteristics to those listed previously for art therapy in general (see Chapter 1, C).

The teenager typically "flees confrontation and is suspicious of any form of adult-driven directives" (Riley, 1999, p. 45). It is crucial for the adolescent in treatment to feel that he has power and control in the client/therapist relationship. Moreover, he needs to feel that it is his free choice if, when and how he addresses issues, and what he wants to share verbally with the adult. In order to avoid confinement by adult rules, adolescents generally like to use their own individualized metaphor (Riley, 1999). Moon (1998) defines "metaphor" as describing "one thing in terms of another. The purpose of this is to shed new light on the character of an object or idea" (p. 9). However, Moon (1998) has a stern warning: the therapist should not label and interpret an adolescent's artwork without getting first a verbal validation by the client. "Just as original creation of an image is a projective interpretation of life on the part of the artist, so too any subsequent attempt to interpret the image is a similar projection on the part of the interpreter" (Moon, 1998, p. 54).

Moon (1998) describes six main themes that frequently arise during an adolescent's art-therapy journey: identity confusion; risk-taking; suicidality; self-loathing; intense anger; and fear of abandonment. Riley (1999) also mentions the extreme narcissism of adolescence: "Focusing on themselves exclusively is one of the mechanisms that fosters this search for identity" (pp. 41–43). "The sense of self is so fragile that confirming to peer group dress codes, musical choices, vocabulary, and hair styles, are all attempts to find some reassurance and identity" (Riley, 1999, p. 43). Art is an ideal mirror in which the teenager, without having to discuss it with adults, can create and reflect his personalized image during the search for his identity. That search, though, can be troubling. For one thing, adolescents tend to take risks out of a sense of grandiosity and omnipotence, thus exhibiting a "disturbing sense of invulnerability and immortality" (Moon, 1998, p. 155) that have to be addressed by the therapist in order to help the teenager avoid self-harm (Moon, 1998). But the therapist also has to keep in mind that "adolescents who avoid experimentation and risk also tend to constrict the evolution of their own independence" (Moon, 1998, p. 155). These are the dynamics the therapist needs to be aware of: Where self-loathing more often than not is verbalized more overtly, suicidal ideation may appear more indirectly in "metaphoric warning signals left by the adolescent for others to find" (Moon, 1998, p. 158). Anger and frustration are common features; adolescents often express these emotions through maladaptive behavior. Warning signs expressed in art or initial forms of mild misbehavior have to be addressed to prevent escalation. Moon (1998) advises art therapists to respond to anger, but not to react to it. Fear of abandonment, finally, may be expressed by adolescents with emotional disturbances and/or corresponding experiences in early childhood. Often fear of abandonment seems to include fear of lack of understanding, fear of retaliation and fear of lack of control and holding by the adult (Moon, 1998).

During his years of working with adolescents, Moon (1998) found that there was a certain pattern through the therapeutic journey. He describes four distinct but overlapping phases: "resistance," "imagining," "immersion" and, finally, "letting go."

The resistance phase reflects the above-mentioned initial difficulties of engaging the adolescent. Moon (1998) describes resistance as "the psychological protection developed by a patient to preserve an inner ego-integrity" (p. 89). He talks about the three main factors that cause this resistance: (1) In most cases the teenager has been forced to come to art therapy, but does not necessarily understand the need for it; (2) adolescents generally mistrust adults, especially authority figures; and (3) the adolescent is hurt in his omnipotence and grandiosity. Moon (1998) lists five recurrent maneuvers of resistance performed by his clients: "The rebel"; "I'm in the In-Crowd/You're in the Out-Crowd"; "Compliant surrender"; "Running away"; and "You're the only one who understands me." "The rebel" tries to defeat the therapeutic structure. By acting out, he tries to disrupt the function of the therapeutic setting. "I'm in the In-Crowd/You're in the Out-Crowd" describes a behavior in which the teenager invests mainly in clique formation with peers. By excluding the therapist from this clique and sabotaging his efforts, the teenager tries to abolish all therapeutic initiatives. In "Compliant surrender" the client shows a behavior in which he complies easily with all the expectations and rules of the therapeutic setting. With this attitude the teenager avoids any kind of confrontation with issues. Needless to say that if such resistances are not addressed and dealt with, the therapy will be without any effect. The "Running away" maneuver has a similar goal. By running away – literally or metaphorically in pictures – the client avoids confrontation through non-participation. Finally, when adolescents use the "You're the only one who understands me" maneuver, "the underlying purpose is to devalue the art therapist, who is then seen as being no different than the patient and therefore of no potential benefit" (Moon, 1998, p. 112).

To this list of resistance maneuvers Linesch (1988) adds a list of defense mechanisms she observed in adolescents' artwork. In a previous chapter, the definition, function, and different manifestations of defense mechanisms typical in adolescence have been listed (Hofmann, 1997; Neinstein, 1991). As an art therapist Linesch (1988) focuses on four things she found in images: (1) Reversal of affect – difficult feelings around an issue are replaced by an adverse feeling (e.g., attachment is replaced by hostility); (2) Increase in narcissism – a distressing and anxiety-provoking feeling is replaced by an increased attachment to oneself; (3) Noncompromise – a "rigid adherence to moral, ethical positions" (Linesch, 1988, p. 20) helps to avoid confrontation with an issue; and (4) Isolation – "involves the separation of affect from content" (Linesch, 1988, p. 22), usually by repressing or displacing the affect to another situation. Linesch (1988) also describes defense mechanisms such as displacement, regression, intellectualization, repression and denial, which have been elaborated on in a previous chapter.

Imagining, the second of the therapeutic phases described by Moon (1998), is characterized by a certain sense of sadness that arises as the adolescent begins to understand the meaning of the previous resistance phase; that means he starts to become aware of his needs. "These needs include a deep longing for support, containment, stability, predictability, and emotional safety" (Moon, 1998, p. 116). "The solid foundation of trust the patient and the art therapist formed as they weathered the resistance phase together provides a powerful base for imagining a different way of being in the world for the adolescent" (Moon, 1998, p. 116).

The third phase, immersion, is where the teenager starts to be "able to connect to his or her inner experiences, and to consistently assume ownership for present emotional and behavioral difficulties" (Moon, 1998, p. 121). Gradually the teen may let go of old, negative self-perceptions and will replace them by new, more positive ones. Ideally he may emerge from this phase with a clearer sense of who he is in this world, with all the positive and negative attributes that go with it.

The last phase, letting go, is also called termination. It is "a period of internalization and consolidation of the gains made during the treatment process" (Moon, 1998, p. 127). It is also a last step of treatment, one in which the adolescent will learn to end an important relationship in a meaningful way, and to transfer newly acquired capabilities into his independent life.

Again I would like to remind the reader to acknowledge caution in using these phase-oriented schemes, since they are rarely linear and chronological (Kuebler-Ross, 1969).

Adolescents are one of the major consumers of psychotherapy. There are variable responses among adolescents sent to treatment. Not all are resistant, and many respond favorably to the presence of a caring, non-judgmental adult. Many adolescents come to treatment for a certain period of time; then they stop it, only to return later. Conflicts around dependence are often demonstrated in this way (Korenblum, 1998).

In the second part of this chapter I will elaborate on what the literature says about medical art therapy. Malchiodi (1999) defines it as "the use of art expression and imagery with individuals who are physically ill, experiencing trauma to the body, or who are undergoing aggressive medical treatment such as surgery or chemotherapy" (p. 13). In a medical setting, art therapy is considered to be an "adjunctive treatment" because patients come to a hospital primarily for medical treatment. But in a mental health care center, where patients come mainly for psychotherapy, art therapy may be part of a primary treatment (Councill, 1993). Art therapy takes advantage of the "art's power to tap inner resources that reduce stress and channel distress, and restore, normalize and humanize what are often inhuman circumstances" (Malchiodi, 1998, p. 30).

The emotional impact of hospitalization, physical illness, and invasive medical treatment on an individual is associated with his cognitive development. In a previous chapter I elaborated on the psychological impact of physical illness on adolescents. Since there is little in the literature about medical art therapy with adolescents, I will briefly focus in this chapter on the psychological impact of physical illness on both those in childhood and those in adulthood.

The younger the child, the less he is able to separate his environment from his self, and to distinguish between reality and fantasy. The older the child and the more sophisticated his thinking, the more he is potentially able to differentiate between external and internal worlds. However, "only in adolescence can the patient have a temporal comprehension of the stages of an illness" (Prager 1993, p. 2).

According to Wadeson (2000), the vulnerability of children to stress depends on six factors: (1) the child's chronological and developmental age as it relates to the ability to understand the illness; (2) responses to previous hospitalizations and separations; (3) emotional support, particularly from the family; (4) coping and communicating skills; (5) cultural definitions of illness and modern medical treatments; and (6) the child's physical condition and the prognosis of the disease. According to Malchiodi (1999), the primary sources of stress in pediatric patients are: (1) separation from parents or caretaker through hospitalization, which results in fear of abandonment and isolation; (2) loss of independence and control; and (3) fear about the incomprehensible situation, especially fears and fantasies about medical procedures, which may cause pain and worries about death. Councill (1993) adds to that list a child's common belief that illness and/or treatment is a punishment for some misdeed or bad thought, which generates feelings of guilt (Malchiodi, 1999). Lusebrink "stated that when a child experiences severe illness or trauma, the fragile ability to separate fact from fantasy is compromised" (Prager 1993, p. 2). Moreover, "trauma, both to the psyche and to the body, is inevitably a part of children's experiences with illness, hospitalization and medical intervention" (Malchiodi 1998, p. 177).

By contrast, the main stress issues of physically ill adults involve struggles with the loss of autonomy, of the loss of control over their lives (Malchiodi, 1998; Malchiodi, 1999). Other big issues include the loss of health; the loss of a functioning body with all its consequences (loss of job, financial problems, changed role within the family dynamics, etc.); and, in many cases, confrontation with death. Consequently, emotional stress for adults revolves primarily around grief and mourning about losses (Landgarten, 1981).

In both children and adults, the above mentioned experiences associated with physical illness result in a negative impact on self-confidence, self-esteem, bodily integrity and body image, and self-identification. The goal of medical art therapy with this population is generally "to initiate and/or maintain a motivation for self-acceptance and adjustment" (Landgarten, 1981). Medical art therapy focuses on helping the individual to gain/maintain a maximum of autonomy within the boundaries of his disability (Landgarten, 1981). It is more about discovering and enhancing strengths, than stressing weaknesses (Malchiodi, 2003).

Both adult and pediatric patients potentially can benefit in many different ways from medical art therapy:

1. According to Landgarten (1981), a patient who is an active participant in art therapy is in full charge of his own decision-making. By making his own choices about art material and theme, he regains some sense of control. An adult cancer patient described her experience as follows: "Painting provided the one control I had over my situation. . . . Doctors controlled my body, but I controlled my soul" (Malchiodi, 1998, p. 172). By creating a tangible piece of art, the ill individual is transformed from a "passive victim of a disease into an active partner in the work of getting well" (Malchiodi, 2003, p. 213). "Symbolically, the art therapy session proves to the patient that dependency (regression due to the need to be taken care of) and independence (taking responsibility) can coexist" (Landgarten, 1981, p. 336). By becoming an active participant in this part of treatment, the patient gains a sense of mastery, which in turns helps to enhance self-confidence and rebuild a sense of self (Malchiodi, 1999).

2. According to Wadeson (2000), "art therapy can provide an important outlet for the ventilation of feelings" (p. 123). By being thrown onto paper, these feelings are "projected externally and magically banned to a certain extent" (Guenter, 2000, p. 11). As discussed in a previous chapter, gaining distance from fears and anxieties by externalizing these feelings, may make them appear less threatening (Farrell Fenton, 2000). "The art work allows patients to distance themselves from painful affect, giving them a chance, metaphorically, to separate

themselves from their disease" (Gabriels, 1988, p. 68; Epping & Willmuth, 1994).

3. As a simple distraction art therapy may help to relieve a person's physical symptoms like pain. Paul Klee, who suffered from Scleroderma, wrote: "Never have I drawn so much nor so intensive. . . . I create in order not to cry" (Malchiodi, 1998, p. 170). Through the creative process the patient gains a sense of normalcy, at least temporarily.

4. Art therapy enhances communication between the patient and his environment. Externalizing problematic feelings not only helps him to explore these emotions from a safe distance, but it also reframes his beliefs about the cause of illness or injury (Malchiodi 1999). Even adults "often have two explanations for their condition, one verbal and one non-verbal" (Malchiodi, 1999, p. 15). The verbal explanation involves a rational recounting based on medical knowledge. The nonverbal explanation, though, is a more personal, maybe even preconscious or unconscious version (Malchiodi, 1999). In order to help the patient adjust to his situation it is important for the healthcare provider to understand the patient's understanding and beliefs about his condition, no matter what age. In addition, art therapy provides information about the patient's coping strategies and resilience, as well as his psychosocial needs (Malchiodi, 1999).

5. Art therapy may also have a psychoeducational component. By providing some medical background information in an appropriate layman's language and offering suitable directives, the art therapist can help his client to understand his disease, including triggering risk factors, requested treatment and so forth. (Gabriels, 1988).

Additional potential benefits for pediatric patients include the following:

6. By virtue of his constant presence and the fact he does not administer medications and painful tests, the art therapist provides the sick child with consistency and continuity in an environment that sees the daily changing of medical staff. This kind of reliable, trusting relationship is crucial for a pediatric patient if he has to cope with separation anxiety and fears of abandonment related to hospitalization (Wadeson, 2000).

7. Art therapy offers a great opportunity to explore a compromised body image (Oppenheim, et al. 1984). By utilizing plain cloth dolls, marker and medical instruments, it has therapeutic value in allowing

the child to change role (Favara-Scacco, et al. 2001). By rehearsing medical procedures in an art therapy setting, the patient gains a sense of control and mastery, which in turns enhances tolerance for pain by controlling fear (Malchiodi, 1999).

8. According to Malchiodi (1999), art therapy enhances resilience in physically ill children. She defines resilience as "the successful adjustment and adaptation to life after experiencing an adverse, hostile, or negative event" (p. 13). "Art expression . . . with pediatric patients is supporting and cultivating psychological resources related to resiliency" (Malchiodi, 1998, p. 19).

9. Listed in a previous paragraph were the potential psychological and somatic trauma in children with hospital experiences. With the increasing numbers of survivors of severe diseases in childhood, there has been a growing body of literature about Post-traumatic Stress Disorder (PTSD) in this population (Malchiodi, 2003). Art therapy can be of important help in dealing with a disorder that is characterized by re-experiencing, avoidance, arousal/hyperarousal symptoms and sleeping problems, all of which are often triggered by minor events that seem to threaten bodily integrity (Malchiodi, 2003).

Additional benefits for adult patients include the following:

10. According to Malchiodi (1999), a patient who opens up through self-expression can help him to understand sources of emotional distress, can help him to resolve conflicts and alleviate trauma, and can help him make grief work more effectively.

11. Malchiodi (1999) states that adult patients may experience transcendence through art, which means getting a sense of "going beyond one's illness and more fully enjoying and experiencing life" (p. 19). She observed how her patients also used art in a transformative way by creating a new sense of who they were. This includes aspects like "discovery of answers to unanswered questions . . . revision of the way one lives life, creation of a new 'post-illness' identity, discovery of a meaning for why one's life has been altered by illness" (Malchiodi 1999, p. 20). In that sense art therapy can enhance personal enrichment (Malchiodi, 1999).

Since families are the main support system for patients, especially for pediatric patients, and because "the experience of illness pervades the whole family system" (Malchiodi, 1998, p. 21), art therapy can be beneficial for the whole family.

During my literature search about medical art therapy with adolescents, I have found only a few articles: one case report about medical art therapy with a diabetic adolescent (Raghuraman, 2000), and several studies with a mixed population of children and adolescents. Gabriels (1988) and Raghuraman (2000) describe medical non-compliance as the main symptom in adolescent patients. Gabriels (1988) validates it as a result of "psychological conflict, resistance to authorities, unconscious death wishes, maladaptive coping styles, poorly developed self-care habits, or conflicting values" (p. 59). In her case report, Raghuraman (2000) describes the autonomy-dependence struggle of her adolescent client, which was exaggerated by the limitations of diabetes. She stresses the importance of giving the patient a sense of mastery and control.

In her article "Art Therapy with Pediatric Cancer Patients: Helping Normal Children Cope with Abnormal Circumstances," Councill (1993) gives an interesting overview of the stages of medical art therapy throughout the course of a disease. As an example, she takes a mixed population of children and adolescents who suffer from cancer. She categorizes the main issues that come up in art therapy in relation to the stages of disease: (1) "Diagnosis and Early Treatment," in which "embarrassment, anger and social withdrawal may accompany the child's sudden loss of self" (Councill, 1993, p. 80). The main issues here are assault on identity, self-esteem, and body image (with typical signs of omission, exaggeration or addition of body parts in figure drawings) (Oppenheim et al., 1984). Denial and withdrawal are often observed defense mechanisms. Besides establishing a trustful working alliance, the main function of art therapy at this stage is to help the patient vent feelings related to initial trauma and humiliation. (2) "Middle Phase of Treatment," besides helping the patient to restore a sense of self, the main function of art therapy at this point is to support "the patient through the long-term stress of treatment" (Councill, 1993, p. 82). Through her patients' drawings, the author observed efforts to create and maintain a new bodily integrity and a sense of self during long periods of "necessary, but traumatic violation of . . . body boundaries" (Councill, 1993, p. 83). In stage (3) "Relapse and Palliative Care," "Anger and isolation may resurface" (Councill, 1993, p. 85). "The power of art to give expression to profound existential themes and the relationship with the art therapist can be a strong support to the patient when words are too difficult either to say or to hear"

(Councill, 1993, p. 85). As mentioned in previous paragraphs these stages are not necessarily linear and chronological.

In his novel *Awakening* Oliver Sacks (1990) summarized the function of art therapy in a wonderful way: "Awakening, basically is a reversal. . . . The patient ceases to feel the presence of the illness and the absence of the world, and comes to feel the absence of his illness and the full presence of the world" (p. 53).

Chapter 2

METHODOLOGY

LOCATION

This retrospective, qualitative, non-randomized study was conducted at the Hemodialysis Unit of a Pediatric Hospital.

POPULATION

My original idea was to work with adolescents who had different kinds of chronic physical diseases. But since most of the chronically sick children are outpatients who come to the hospital on a more or less irregular basis for weekly or monthly appointments, I realized that, in order to get more permanent clients, I would have to concentrate on patients with end-stage renal failure in need of dialysis. This population seemed to be the only group that had a regular treatment schedule but were still well enough to be able to draw.

After making contact with the head of Nephrology, I was introduced to the adolescents on the Hemodialysis Unit and their parents by their social worker. The criteria of exclusion: children aged less than 12 years and older than 18 years. Finally, I introduced myself and the function of art therapy to 13 adolescents – 8 males and 5 females. Participation in art therapy was voluntary for all of the unit's teenagers. Five of them (four boys and one girl) declared no interest right away; one boy dropped out after a trial of three sessions. The clients I saw for less than five sessions were not included in this study due to lack of information. In the end, I worked with 7 adolescents over a period of 10 months (four of them for the whole period, three of them on a short-term basis due to their later admission to the unit). I included all seven clients in this case study research.

All of the adolescents involved in the study came from different sociocultural (three Asians, three Caucasians, one African) and religious (three Christians, two Hindus, one Muslim, one Buddhist) backgrounds. The age range of the four long-term cases (two boys, two girls) was between twelve and sixteen years (mean age 13.5 years); the range for the short-term cases (one boy, two girls) was between thirteen and seventeen years (mean age 15 years). Therefore, they were all at various stages of development.

None of the clients had additional psychotherapy, but they all had their own personal social worker meeting with them on a regular base once a week. None of the clients was on any kind of psychoactive medication, but they had multiple medications in relation to their renal failure (steroids, antihypertensive medication, etc.). They all were diagnosed with end-stage renal failure in need for any kind of kidney replacement therapy; none of them was known to have a preexisting mental health disorder according to the DSM IV criteria.

INDEPENDENT VARIABLES

None of the adolescents involved in the study knew the long-term effects of their illness. Nor did they know what the duration of their stay at the unit would be. As a result, one of the short-term girls, who was initially planned for hemodialysis, switched to Peritoneal Dialysis right at the beginning and dropped out of the program after a few sessions. This kind of dialysis is done at home, and the patient has to show up on a more or less regular base for bloodwork once or twice a month. When this teenage girl was physically stabilized enough she did not want to continue with art therapy. One short-term boy was transplanted after two hemodialysis treatments (with his brother as organ donor) and attended the art therapy program for the time he had to stay at the hospital after surgery (about two months). One of the male long-term clients was transplanted after three months of art therapy and decided to continue until the end of the program at the end.

Medical diagnosis leading to end-stage renal failure were:

- Two congenital malformations (one girl, one boy, both short-term)

- One steroid resistant glomerulonephritis (male long-term client) with onset of disease between ages five and six
- One nephrotic syndrome (female short-term client) with onset of disease also between ages five and six
- Two rheumatologic syndromes involving the kidneys (two female long-term clients) developed over the past three years
- One unknown (male long-term client)

Setting

Since these adolescents spend a large part of their lives in hospital sitting on a chair, connected to their hemodialysis machine with a central venous line, for three to four hours, three to four times a week, without any kind of holidays, I quickly understood that they were – understandably – not willing to spend extra time for art therapy at the hospital. So I decided to work with them while they were sitting at their machines. But that meant getting accustomed to a semi-open environment. Therefore, the art therapy sessions took place in a big room with four hemodialysis machines running parallel at a time. Having a private, intimate space where I could guarantee 100 percent confidentiality was out of the question – due, for example, to the presence of nurses who, appropriately, were performing compulsory constant surveillance (monitoring, blood pressure, etc.). However, I quickly realized that this setting was more distracting for me than it was to my clients, because to them it was part of their "normal" life. Nevertheless, I think this kind of special setting has to be kept in mind in relation to their disclosures during a session.

At a certain point I considered group art therapy. But I decided that since the adolescents could not really interact with one another given that each was attached to his proper machine, group work was not appropriate.

Procedure

An "insight-oriented art therapy" in Wadeson's (1987) terms is not appropriate for this population due to the uncertainty concerning the outcome of their illness and treatment and the fluctuation in their physical symptoms. These adolescents are dealing primarily with physical crises and are not looking for Art Psychotherapy. Therefore, I have chosen to follow a "client-centered therapy model" in

Wadeson's (1980) terms, one in which the therapist provides a non-threatening and non-judgmental environment for the client. The goal is to encourage the client to express himself in his own way at his own pace. I applied a mainly non-directive, spontaneous approach of art therapy in order to enhance the opportunities for the children, who generally experience a lot of external control, to make their own choices and decisions. Rarely, and only on the client's request, would I offer a choice of very open directives (e.g., the tree drawing, the bridge drawing, etc.). In these instances, I would always give the children the option to eventually reject these suggestions. I never offered interpretations of art products, but rather encouraged the client to have a final verbal processing, or "free associations," at the end of the session.

At the beginning of the art therapy program the termination date was fixed – the end of the school term. I worked at the facility for 10 months, and tried to meet with each client at least once a week. Mondays, Wednesdays and Fridays were the hemodialysis days. I tried to be as flexible as possible in offering additional opportunities for make-up sessions whenever a session had to be skipped for medical reasons. The criteria to interrupt or skip a session were: (1) medical and/or emergency reason; or (2) the client's own wish for whatever reason. In general, the sessions lasted for about 60 minutes. Sometimes, though, we had to stop sooner because of the above-mentioned reasons, or extend a session because the client was in high spirits and wanted to work longer and make-up for previous, shorter sessions. I tried to be as flexible as possible, with the idea of giving back to this population as much control as possible.

The mean number of sessions was 36.75 (with a range from 27 to 48) for the long-term group, and 7.3 (with a range from 5 to 11) for the short-term group.

Materials

I offered paint, pencil, pencil crayons, oil and chalk pastels, markers, clay and collage material (glue, found images of magazines, beads, feathers, pipe cleaners, etc.).

Gathering of Data

The collection of the material happened mainly through my own therapy notes completed after each session plus the art products, meetings and discussions with my supervisor, and whatever parents told me regarding the diagnosis. The questions I was looking for, are concerning tasks characterizing the development of adolescence: (1) achievement of independence from parents, (2) exploration and finally adoption of peer codes and lifestyles, (3) awareness and acceptance of body image, and finally (4) establishing sexual, ego, vocational and moral identities.

Color Plate Section

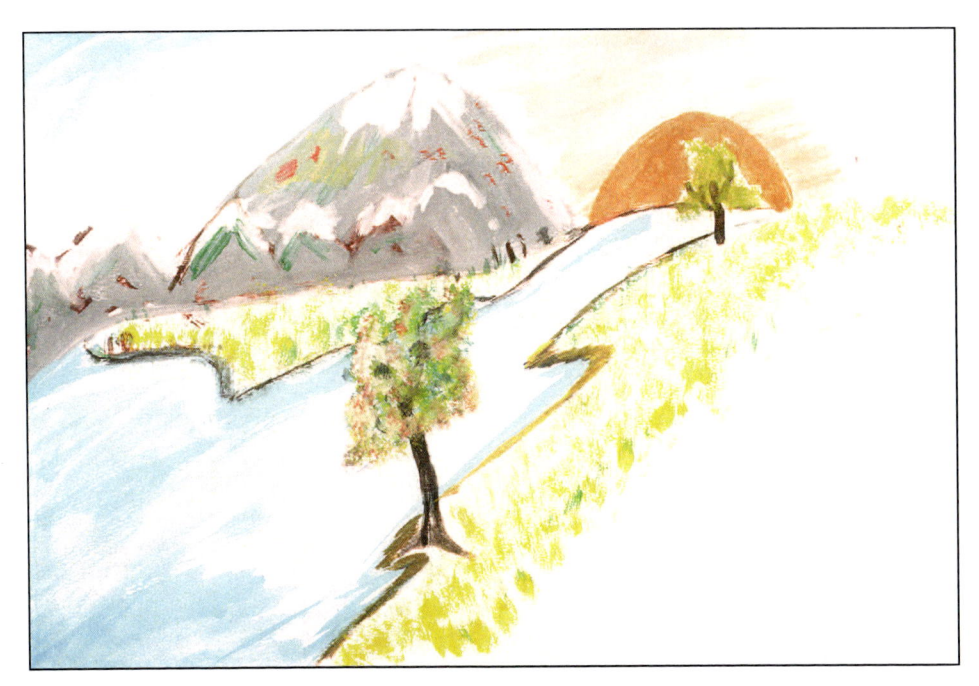

Plate 1. *A Landscape*, watercolor by Abdul, 16 years.

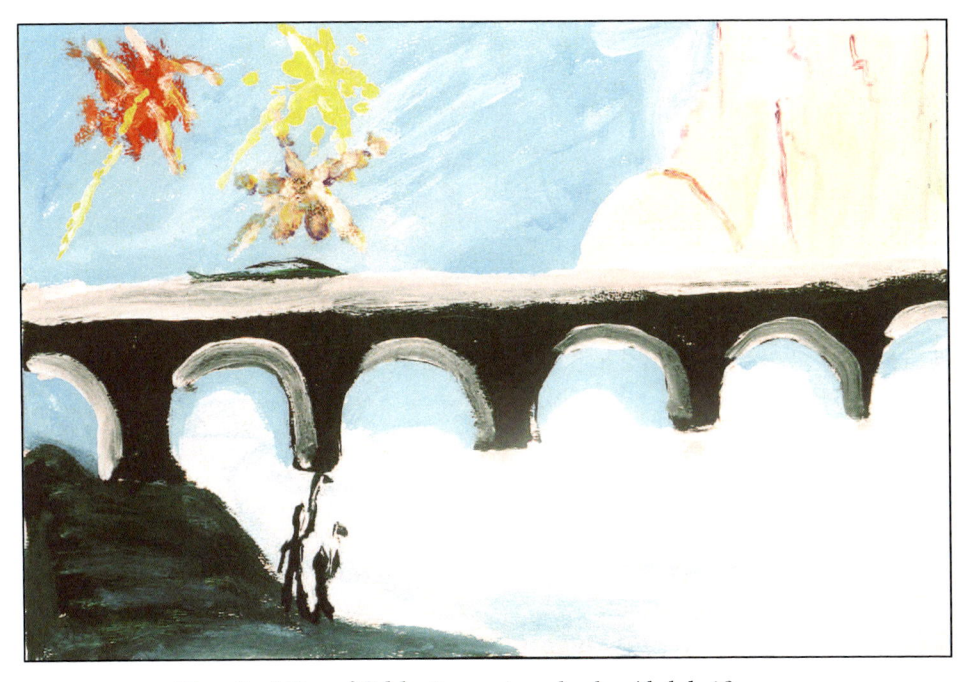

Plate 2. *A Day of Celebration*, watercolor by Abdul, 16 years.

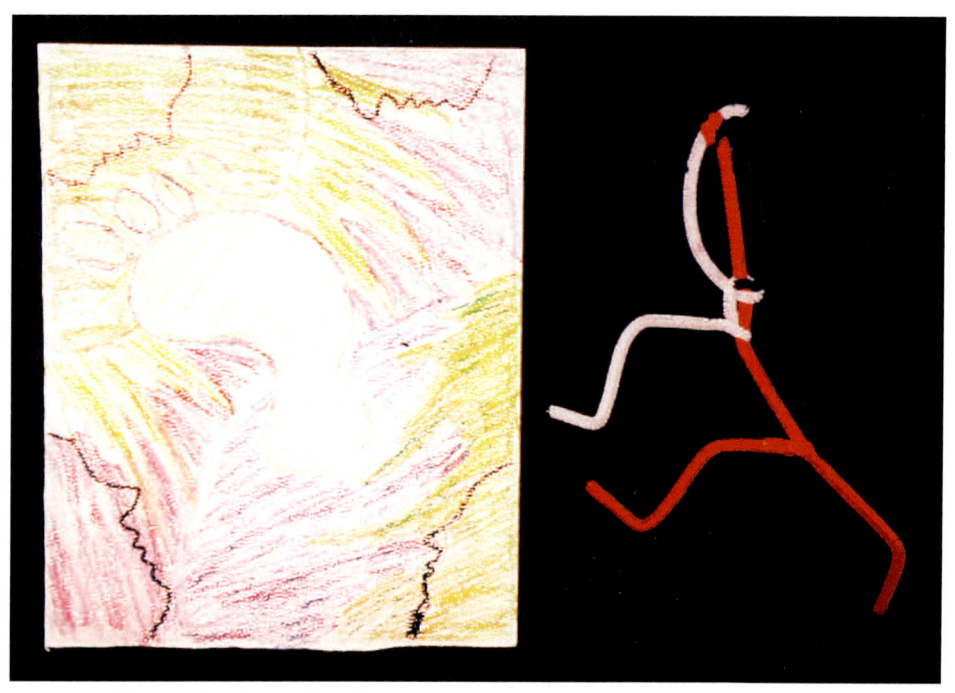

Plate 3. *The Green Step Towards the Sun*, oil pastels by Abdul, 16 years.

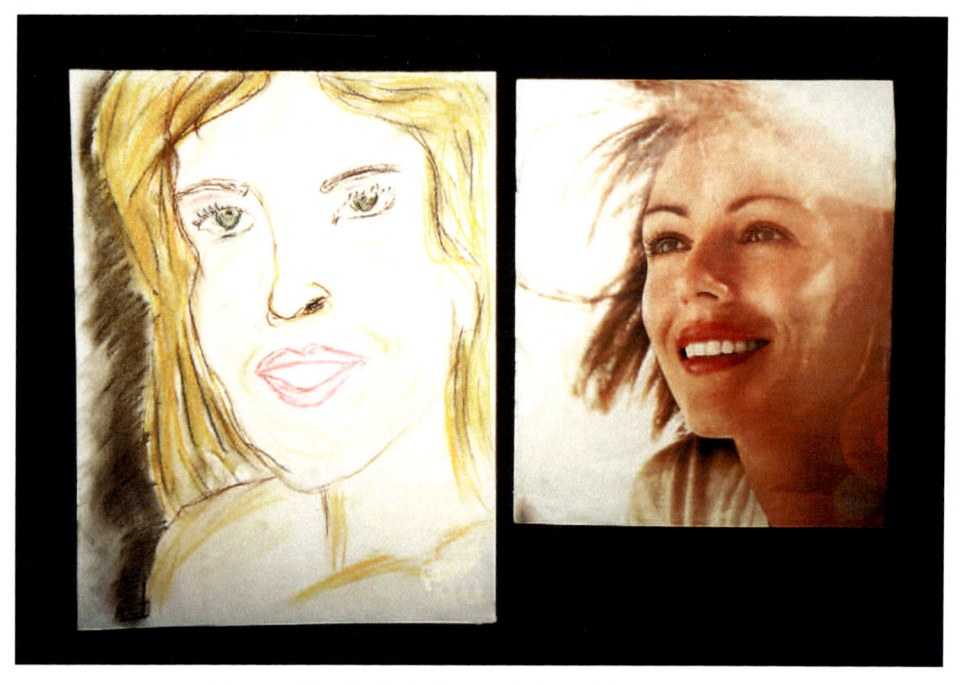

Plate 4. Untitled, chalk pastels by Abdul, 16 years.

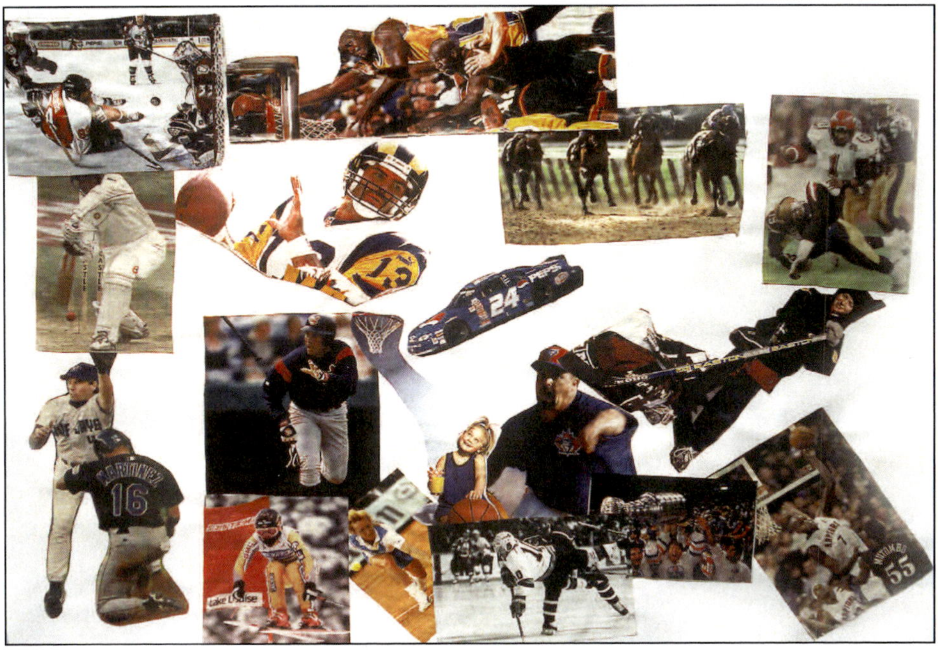

Plate 5. *Sports*, collage by Jayson, 13 years.

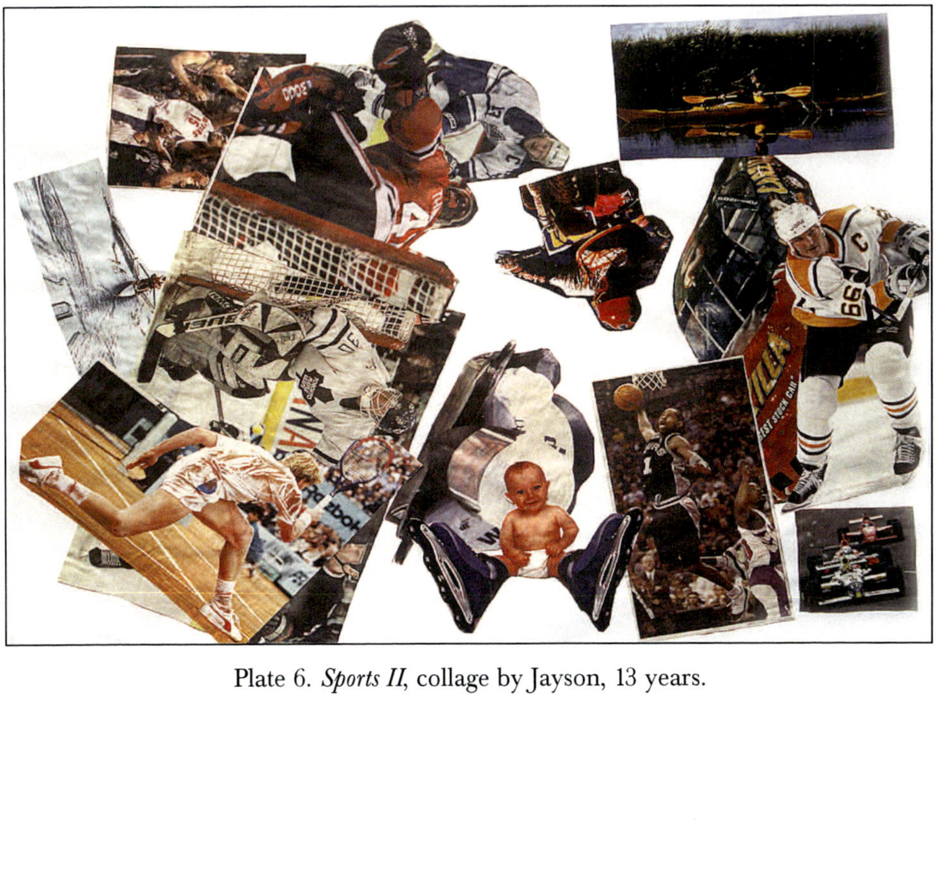

Plate 6. *Sports II*, collage by Jayson, 13 years.

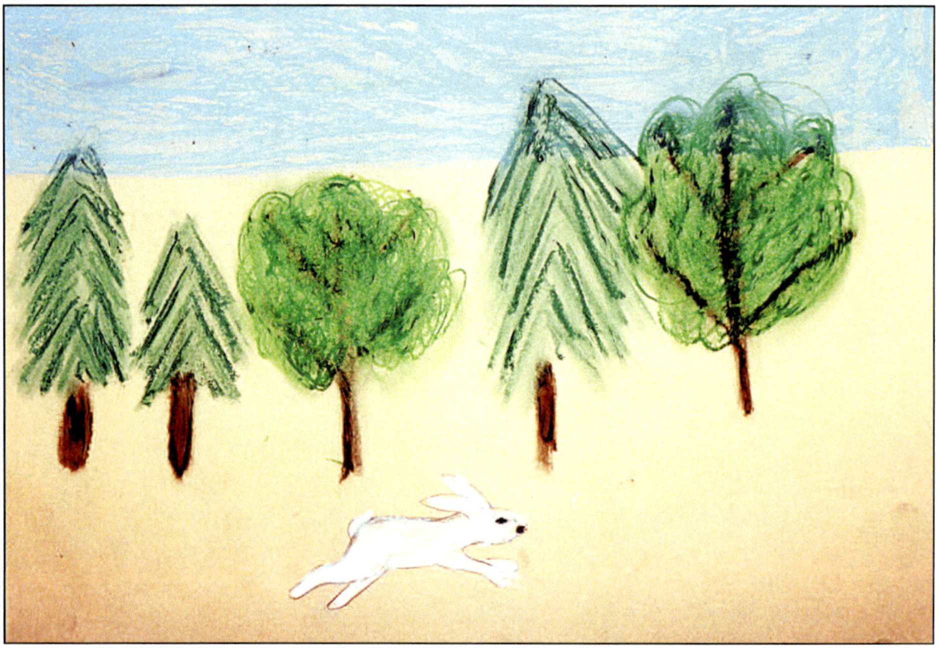

Plate 7. *My White Rabbit*, oil pastels by Katja, 12 years.

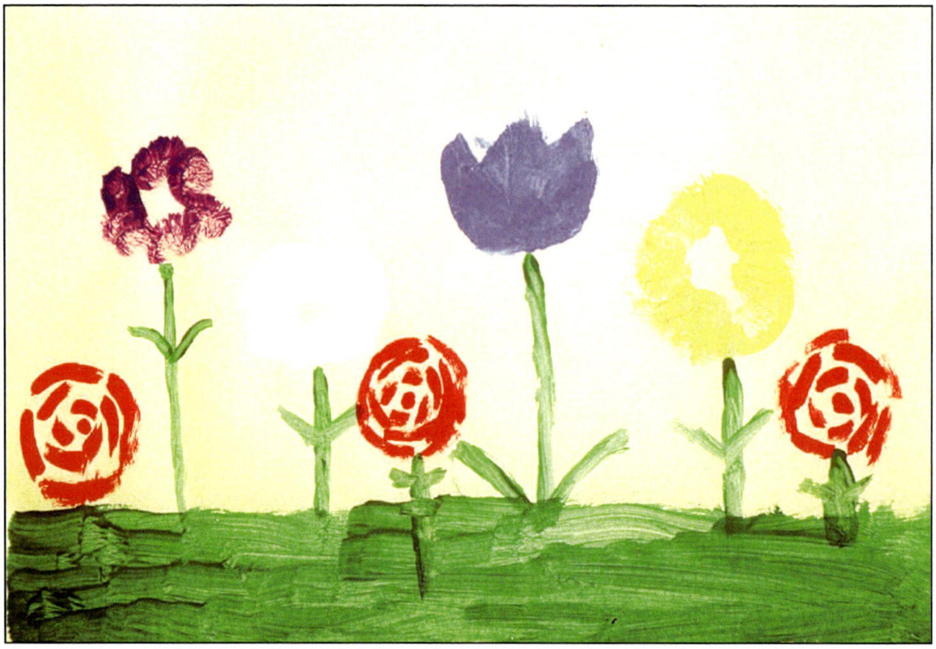

Plate 8. *Spring Flowers*, watercolor by Katja, 12 years.

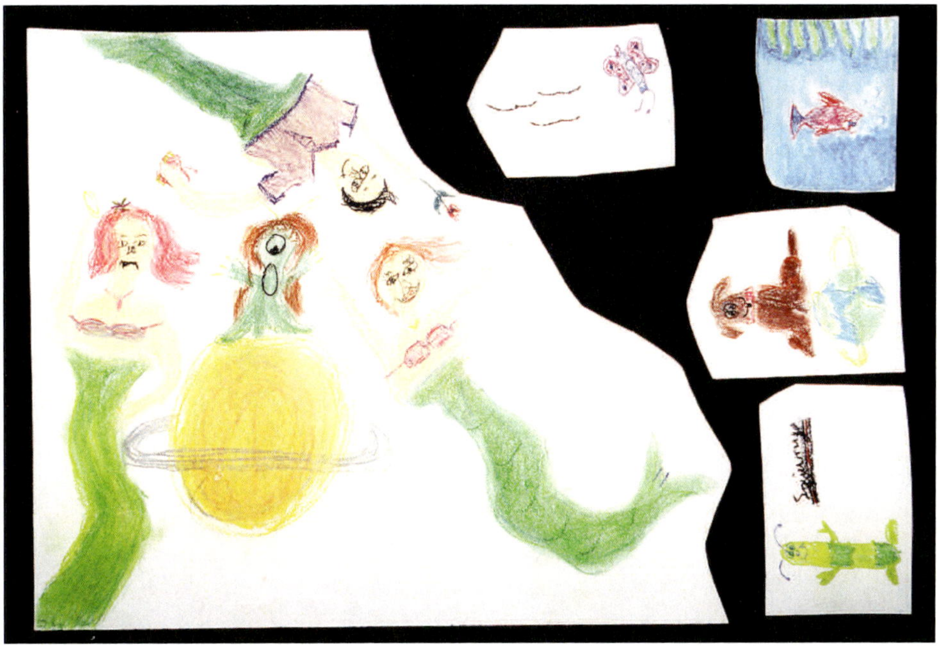

Plate 9. Untitled, chalk pastels by Nadja, 13 years.

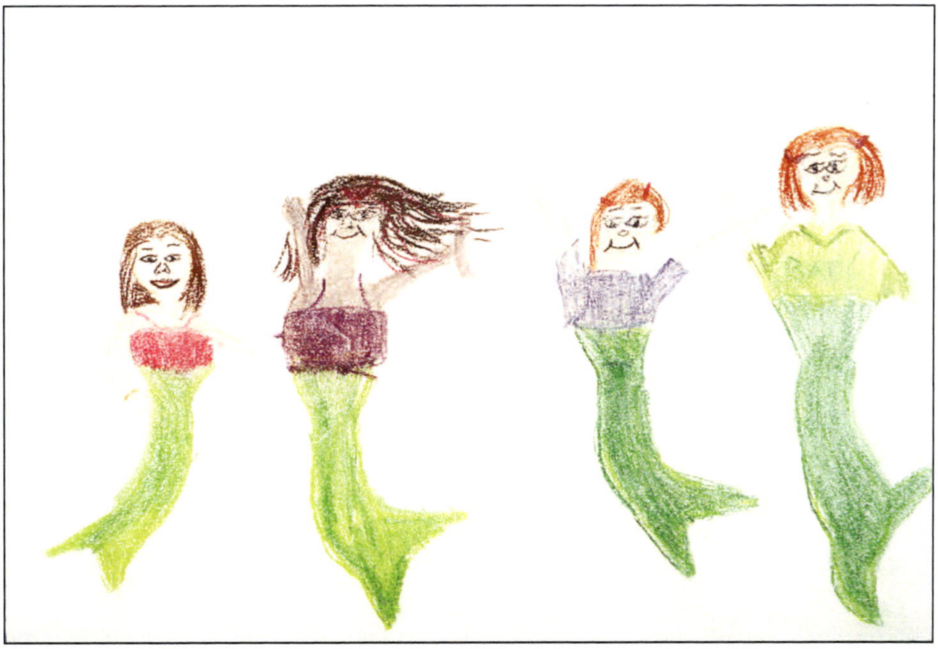

Plate 10. *Family Portrait*, chalk pastels by Nadja, 13 years.

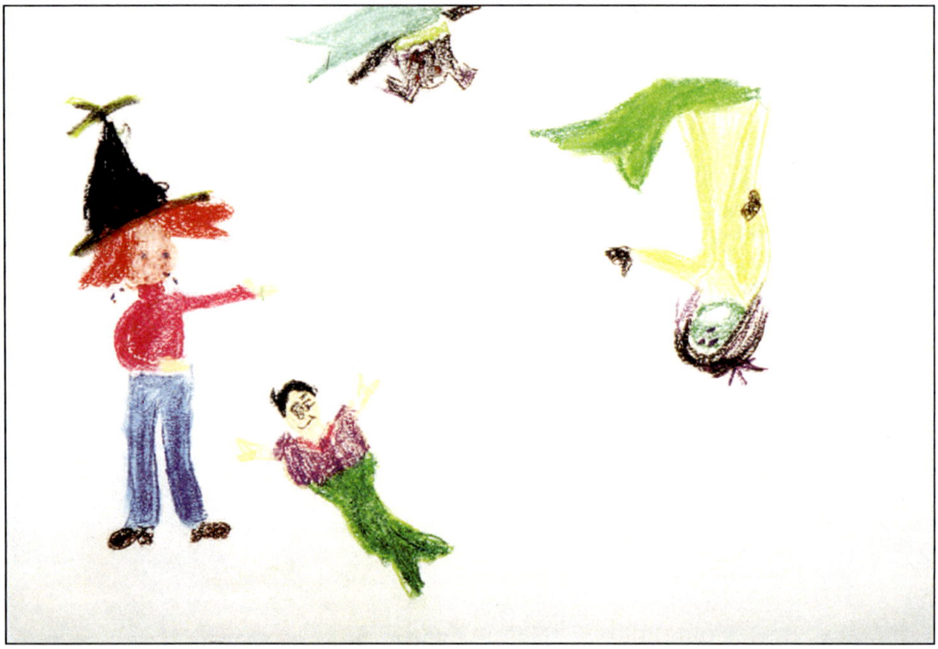

Plate 11. *Mark's Story,* chalk pastels Nadja, 13 years.

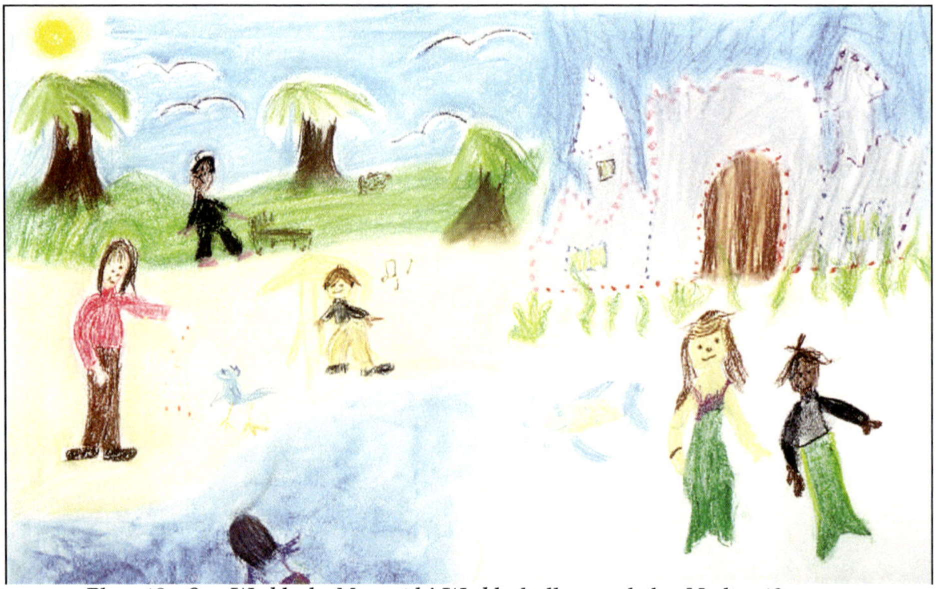

Plate 12. *Our World, the Mermaids' World,* chalk pastels by Nadja, 13 years.

Chapter 3

CASE HISTORIES AND ARTWORK

In order to protect their personal privacy I have changed the names of all the clients discussed below. But for the purposes of better understanding their actions and reactions, I have kept their respective age, gender and sociocultural background.

Since the outcome of an art therapy course is dependent on the duration of treatment – as well as the personalities of client and therapist, sociocultural backgrounds, developmental maturity, and so forth. – I have subdivided my seven cases into two groups: a short-term treatment group of three adolescents (with five to eleven sessions, mean 7.3 sessions) and a long-term treatment group of four (with 27 to 48 sessions, mean 36.75 sessions).

The clients were informed and agreed with the use of their picture for this work. In this chapter I will add thoughts and associations given by the client about their actual artwork, including my own immediate reactions to the piece, directly to the particular print. More general use of and reaction to the art therapy process I am going to summarize for each client in Chapter 4 (discussion).

A. SHORT-TERM TREATMENT GROUP

1. Emma, Female, 13 Years

Description of the Client

Emma is a thirteen-year-old Caucasian girl of Polish origin. Her long blonde hair was bound into a ponytail most of the time. She is of short and chubby stature, most likely due to her chronic renal conditions, which demanded long-term steroid treatment. Physically she appeared to be just entering puberty since she exhibited few secondary female features.

From the very beginning she was open, friendly and communicative, and she seemed to be very interested in doing art. Her interaction with me, including conversation, showed a well-balanced pattern of offering information about herself and asking questions about me. She always performed with a well-controlled, almost guarded manner, and was always cooperative, never questioning anything. She had clear ideas about her art projects and was able to communicate her wishes in an appropriate way. In her I often saw a well-educated young adult with rational thinking who often kept her real feelings well- hidden.

Social History

Emma was the oldest of three children of Polish immigrants. With her parents, she immigrated when she was seven years old. Her six-year-old brother was the first child of the family who was born in North America. Her younger sister was just about two weeks old when I first met Emma. With some underlying bitterness in her voice Emma let me know that only now, after the birth of the third child, there was some justification for her mother to stay at home with the children. "I would have needed her as well with my illness," she revealed one day. It was the only time I could feel her own needs. Her mother had been working as a hairdresser; her father is a construction worker. The family's closest relatives still live in Poland.

Emma was a good student in grade eight, loved to go to school and apparently had a lot of good friends. Due to her frequent absences from school, she was not sure if she would make it into grade nine and would therefore miss her friends terribly. She offered me all this information without showing any emotions.

Medical History

At the age of five years – still back home in Poland – Emma developed a Nephrotic Syndrome, a disease of unknown cause but one brought on by a multiple of suspected triggering mechanisms. Nephrotic Syndrome is characterized by a leakage of protein through the kidney's filter with otherwise intact kidney functions. It is a well-known problem in younger children, with usually a benign prognosis under steroid treatment. In Emma's case the disease did not respond to the therapy and, over the years, she developed an uncontrollable loss of protein through her kidneys to the point of making daily intravenous protein substitution necessary. When hypertension worsened her situation, she had to have both kidneys removed, which made her dependent on kidney replacement therapy. Initially postoperative hemodialysis was planned. As a result, Emma and her family were prepared appropriately and introduced to the hemodialysis team and the other patients. But it was impossible to install a working central venous line. Therefore, the doctors had to urgently switch her to peritoneal dialysis and implant a tube into her abdominal cavity. The change in treatment meant that the family needed to reorganize the plumbing in their house since peritoneal dialysis is done at home. It also meant a big change in training, especially for Emma and her mother, since they now had to take full responsibility for the treatment. As part of the training Emma was hospitalized for about three weeks so that her mother could come into the hospital on a daily basis so she could practice what needed to be done in a monitored environment. That was the period in which I met them, and started to work with Emma.

Art Therapy Process and Artwork

When we started to work together the idea was to establish a trustful working alliance while Emma was hospitalized, and then to continue art therapy on a weekly basis as an outpatient when she had to come to the hospital to check her blood once a week. Mother and daughter agreed with this procedure (unfortunately, I never had the honor of meeting the father).

After the introduction and demonstration of the available art materials, Emma immediately wanted to start making a big collage on a white piece of paper (Figure 3.1: "Wild Animals," collage by Emma, 13 years). The theme was animals because she loved animals and wanted to become a veterinarian. For the first three sessions she concentrated on the same collage, talked a lot and addressed many issues, many of them totally unrelated to her art piece. They included discussions of: (1) her original homeland, Poland, where she started taking lessons in horseback riding and where she visited a zoo; she also talked about some recipes for Polish specialties; (2) her school, where she attended grade eight as a good student and where she had many good friends she'd miss if she failed to be promoted to grade nine. (3) Her family, especially her new sister, who was the reason her mother planned to give up working so she could stay at home with the children; and (4) my other art therapy clients on the hemodialysis unit; after she realized that her room was on the other side of the inner court, just opposite to the hemodialysis unit, and that she could observe the children sitting on their machines from her bed, she started to wonder about the techniques they were using and the themes they were elaborating in their art therapy with me.

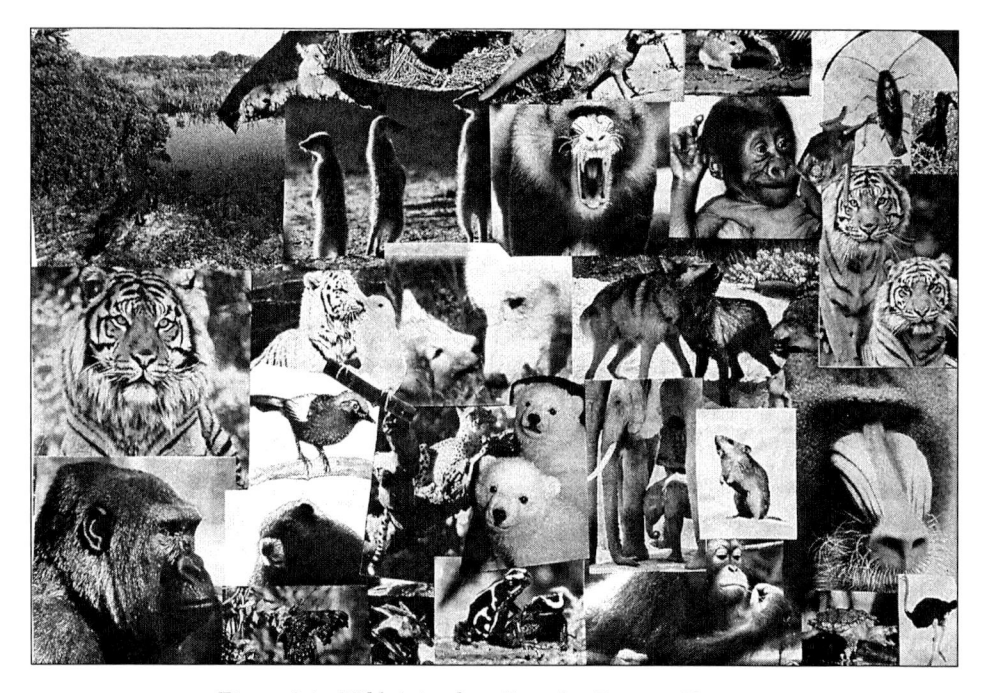

Figure 3.1. *Wild Animals*, collage by Emma, 13 years.

Right from the beginning her main concern in relation to her collage was to close all the gaps between the pictures, absolutely avoiding any blank paper shining through. This was an ongoing preoccupation throughout the time she was working on her collage. It was like an obsession – she was anxious to find smaller and smaller images to fill in the space, and finally asked for creative ideas to cover the spots that were definitely too small for pictures. Markers brought a big relief to her anxiety. At the beginning of her art-making process, Emma seemed to concentrate more on the content of the photographs – she was very conscious of how she chose the animals. Later on, however, she was more concerned about how to find images small enough to fit into tiny gaps, apparently regardless of the content of the image.

By the end of the third session she seemed to be satisfied with her piece, which now showed a well-sealed surface with overlapping photographs and marker dots. Her obsessive behavior to close the smallest-possible gap was striking. The tendency to fill every single square centimeter of a piece of paper is known in anxious, very insecure children, who try to avoid any kind of unpredictibilities by not leaving open choices for the fantasy, and who need to keep everything under control in order to avoid surprises (Oster & Gould, 1987). Another explanation could be that it was a metaphoric self-portrait, one in which she desperately tried to make the piece as complete and perfect as possible in order to reverse her body image of imperfection and defectiveness. Or was it a reflection of her very tight upbringing not leaving her any freedom to be a child?

There was, however, another notable feature in this work: her attempts to put two animals of the same species in relation to each other. In the beginning she chose photographs of couples of the same animals (e.g., polar bears, wolves, tigers, elephants, frogs, etc.). Later, she would overlap single animals onto a previously glued photograph (e.g., two birds, two tigers, etc.). Often it would be an adult and a young animal. She never made comments about her choices of animals, nor wanted to give me any associations about her collage. Instead she told me about her mother finally being allowed to stay at home with the children only after the birth of her little sister. I asked her how she felt about that, and her answer was: "Oh, I'm happy to have her back. I would have needed her, too, when I was a small child back home with my disease." Making all sorts of animal couples in her collage was perhaps the metaphoric expression of her need for closeness, emotional nourishment and support; maybe also of her need for being allowed to still be a child. Right from the beginning I sensed in Emma that she exhibited the behavior of a small adult, someone who appeared overwhelmed by the burden of responsibility she had within her family.

For the third session, Emma wanted to close it by decorating the cover of her portfolio. She glued a single photograph with the head of a howling wolf in the centre of the big cover, as if giving expression to a sad loneliness, and added: "I don't want to write my name onto the cover. The two of us will know whose work this is. I don't want people to know it's mine." She did not offer further associations to the wolf or her piece of art.

At the beginning of the fourth session she announced that she might be discharged by the end of the week, and that she would like to try something new.

She decided to work in clay and to make a sculpture for her new room at home (Figure 3.2: "Bud of a Flower," clay sculpture by Emma, 13 years). Carefully she made a wide-open flower with a thick stem, but then decided to close it tightly into a bud, as if she wanted to keep a secret inside. During the fifth – and, as I learned later, our last – session she painted her flower and asked for a creative idea in order to make leaves. When she had a final, satisfied look at her finished piece, she commented: "That's strange. It looks like a human figure, with open arms." I had a similar association: a child who opens her arms to be taken into a beloved person's arms, or who would like to be hugged. She agreed with me, and quickly asked for a box to protect it. This still young flower, which seemed to hold in some important secret and which, despite its thick stem, needed to be stabilized on popsicle sticks, was perhaps a kind of metaphoric self-portrait of Emma.

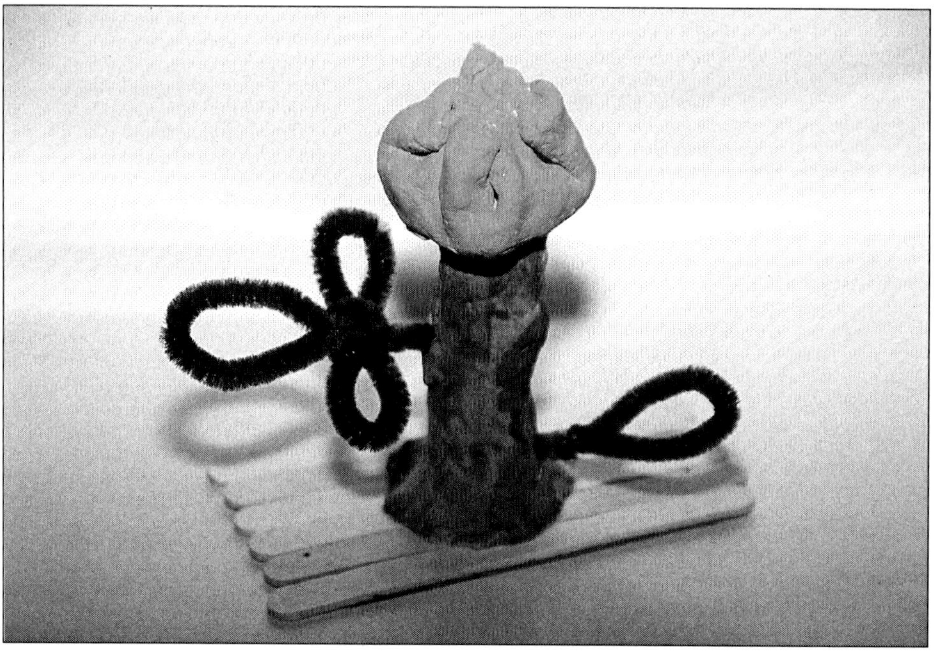

Figure 3.2. *Bud of a Flower*, clay sculpture by Emma, 13 years.

After she became an outpatient I tried several times to meet with her and to arrange further art therapy sessions. Emma and her mother seemed to avoid me, and without the help of the coordinating nurse I would have never seen them again. At that very last meeting the mother told me that Emma did not want to continue to work with me. The mother told me that at Emma's age one is too busy at school, and does not have extra time to spend at the hospital. As for Emma, she was physically present but seemed to be emotionally absent, impossible to reach for me, as if shut off. I was wondering whether the decision to stop art therapy was really hers, considering the engagement she showed during the sessions. In a last attempt I tried to convince the mother of the benefits for Emma, but her decision was made. Was her biggest concern to lose her "good girl" who was so good in taking over responsibilities?

SUMMARY

Thirteen-year-old Emma with her behavior of a well-educated adult was very well able to connect with me, always keeping her feeling well under control. During the whole time we spent together she was involved in her art, and seemed to enjoy the process. Not only her artwork but also her behavior reflected her need for peer contacts. Often I had the feeling she was using me as a connection to the world outside of her family, especially to other physically ill adolescents, mainly kidney patients. Her artwork expressed tension and anxiety, as well as loneliness, as a result of her being overwhelmed by the responsibility as the family's "good girl." Unfortunately, we did not have enough time together, to overcome the initial phase of resistance, and to develop a trustful working alliance.

2. Joan, Female, 17 Years

Description of the Client

Joan is a seventeen-year-old Caucasian girl. Her long blonde curled hair was always pulled back in a thick braid. She had the physical size of an eight-year-old, but the pubertal development of a fifteen-year-old with some secondary female sexual features. As part of herself she always pulled a little cart that held a bottle of compressed oxygen. Her body had grown very asymmetrically and distorted. Due to her scoliotic back she was very restricted in movements; but the few movements she was able to do (including walking and running) were surprisingly dexterous. Her main handicap (and part of her congenital syndrome) was a fused and stiff neck, which resulted in her head being bent asymmetrically to her left shoulder and her face turned to the left side. Taken together, the result was a grotesque disfigurement of her face (left eye much lower then the right, crooked nose and mouth, deformation of left lower jaw with overlapping teeth, etc.). At first sight, one might think she was a human being who couldn't communicate at all. But she would teach me different.

From the very beginning Joan was open and friendly, and was communicative without being overly talkative. Although her facial features made it difficult for me to understand her, she loved to tell me about her family and her social environment. However, she never asked me anything about myself or the other children in therapy. She usually was in an even or good mood, and seemed to be happy in her own small world. Although she was very limited in her possibilities due to her restricted mobility, she showed a balanced behavior of trying to help herself and look for assistance. She was able to ask for help in a natural and self-evident way. Often I found myself jumping in with a helping gesture too fast. On these occasions she was able to push me back softly but firmly, without showing signs of being hurt or being humiliated. Although the referring social worker told me that Joan had the intelligence of a nine-year-old, I thought her emotional maturity was much more advanced and almost age appropriate.

Social History

Joan was a well-integrated and average student in grade 10 of a special aid class. She loved to go to school, had a lot of good friends and a very active social life outside her family.

Joan was the oldest of three children. She has a ten-year-old sister and an eight-year-old brother. Her mother is a housewife and her father an employee at a local wine and liquor store. They are humble, uncomplicated and nice people who live in their own house and own a cottage in the country. The family seemed to be very supportive of Joan, and she appears to be well-embedded in an extended family system. Of special importance is the family of Joan's aunt on her mother's side, with two cousins: Ruby, ten years of age, and Andrew, fourteen years of age. They are all practicing Christians and very active in their religious community.

Medical History

After a normal pregnancy and delivery, to the big surprise of everybody, Joan was born with Klippel-Feil Syndrome: a malformation syndrome in which the vertebra of the neck, sometimes including the upper thoracic spine, are fused and immobilized. Therefore, Joan was unable to move her head as a congenital condition. As a consequence she developed a severe scoliosis with consecutive restricted lung disease, which made her chronically dependent on oxygen. As a consequence of her lung disease she had a so-called cor pulmonale with restricted function. As a further complication of her lung disease she developed sleep apnea syndrome, a condition in which the patient does not breathe sufficiently in deep sleep and therefore needs to be put on a home respirator at night. Due to her asymmetrically fixed neck spine, her head and face grew asymmetrically as well. In association with the skeletal malformation, Joan had congenital dysplastic kidneys, which over the years had gradually given up their function to the point that, at age seventeen, kidney replacement therapy was necessary.

Six months after the end of the art therapy program, I heard that Joan's kidney transplant was successful and that, despite her severe impairment, her recovery went extremely well.

Art Therapy Process and Artwork

I started to work with Joan when she had begun hemodialysis. Due to her embarrassing appearance and the difficulty they had in understanding her, the nurses were not too interested in entertaining Joan during the dialysis. Once she was hooked up to her machine, she was left pretty much on her own, and would spend her time watching TV. When asked by the social worker if I could work with Joan, I was hesitant, knowing that there were only about twelve weeks left in my program. I decided to inform her and her mother about the upcoming closing, and to let Joan decide whether she wanted to participate. She did. So when we started to work together it was with the idea of a temporary therapy.

After the introduction and demonstration of the available art material, Joan immediately wanted to decorate the cover of her folder with a drawing. While she was drawing with a pencil, she told me about her family and its members, including her dogs, about her school and her church. Whatever she told me found its way as an image onto paper; whatever she drew she labeled in written words. These were the two typical features of her drawings throughout the art therapy program.

During the first two sessions Joan introduced me to her surrounding world, adding one drawing of her big blue house with mailbox, one of her cottage and van, and one of her entire family (Figure 3.3: "My Family," drawing by Joan, 17 years). To her family with mom, dad, David, herself and Victoria, she added her two cousins, Ruby and Andrew, and her two dogs, Harley and Angel, again labeling all members. While she was working she told me mainly about the two dogs she very much loved, and her cousin Andrew with whom she spends a lot of time playing computer games. Sharing a cottage Joan's family and her mom's sister's family spend a lot of time together. The way she talked about her family gave me the sense of a well-functioning and supportive family dynamic. Although nobody was really grounded – the figures all seemed to free-float in space – Joan's figure appeared well-embedded in the middle of her family, and all family members apparently were of the same importance (same size, similar features, same distances between figures, etc.). Her drawing confirmed my assumption (after having met her mother and her siblings) about a supportive family.

In our third session she decided to try something new and to work in clay (Figure 3.4: "Me and Andrew," clay sculpture by Joan, 17 years). After an initial struggle with the material, she quickly developed problem-solving strategies and then moved on to focusing on her main theme: the human body. While she was exploring the size and position of the head and the length and gestures of the limbs, she told me about her favorite cousin, Andrew, who was 14 years old. Like the two clay stick figures she was making, she and Andrew seemed to be very close, and to spend a lot of time together – playing computer games was their favorite pastime. While her stick figure drawings seemed to be created casually, with her clay figures she tried to get the individual features as correct as possible. Finally, she was satisfied and declared that she was the figure on the right side, whereas Andrew was represented by the left one.

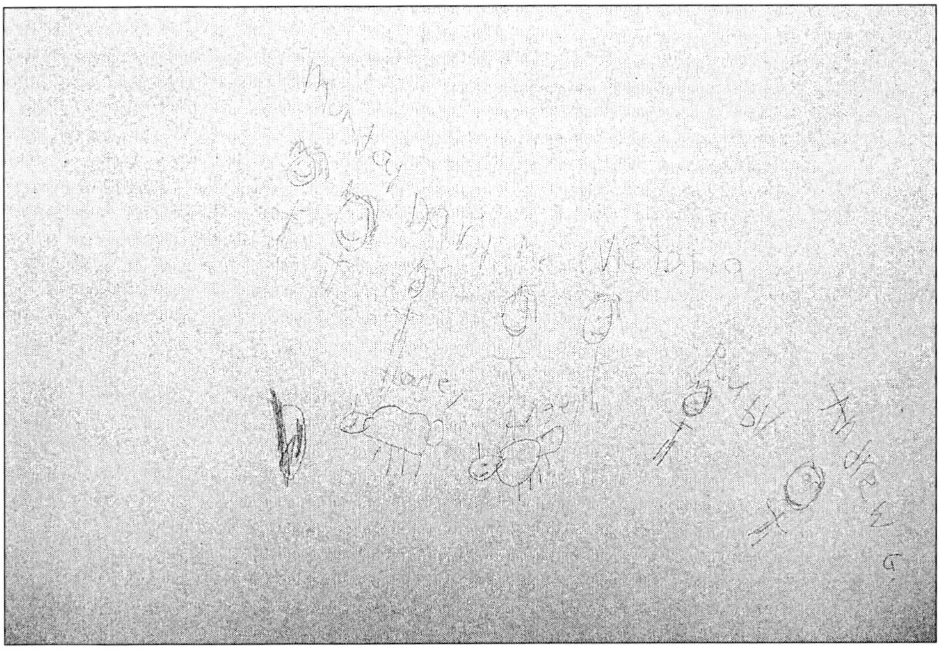

Case Histories and Artwork 61

Figure 3.3. *My Family*, drawing by Joan, 17 years.

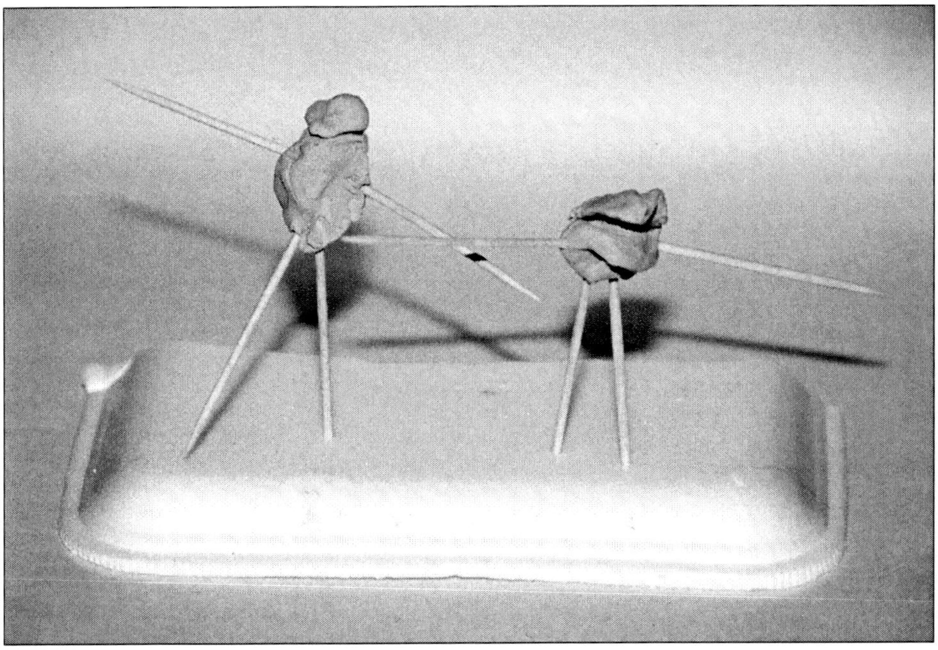

Figure 3.4. *Me and Andrew*, clay sculpture by Joan, 17 years.

During the fourth session she was more irritable and unsettled, but rejected my comment about this observation. She decided to make some pencil drawings, and ended up making one that portrayed her entering the hospital, and one that showed her standing in front of her church with her house in the background (Figure 3.5: "My House and My Church," drawing by Joan, 17 years).

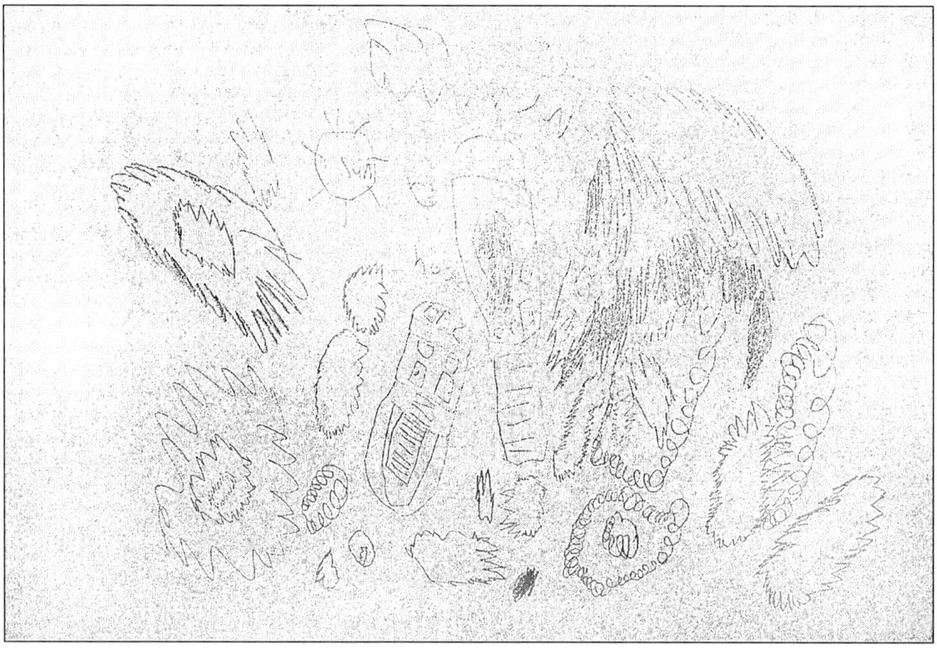

Figure 3.5. *My House and My Church*, drawing by Joan, 17 years.

While she usually worked in a well-controlled and even way, that day her movements appeared fast and almost aimless. She worked quickly and, aside from technical comments related to the picture, talked little.

That day both her drawings showed similar striking features: After having drawn and labeled the main items, she started to add a lot of black clouds and dark bushes. During the course of the art-making process the clouds became darker, the bushes denser and denser, almost suffocating her figure until, finally, her figure was totally invisible and lost in a forest. For the whole time she did not talk spontaneously, nor did she give any associations. I asked her how she was feeling, and got a neutral, apparently uninvolved answer: "Okay."

When she added the same striking features to the second drawing with the hospital, I made a comment about how threatening the mood of this picture was; I tried to investigate her feelings around hospital and disease. "I'm okay at the hospital," was her brief answer. But after a while she started to tell me how her kidneys gradually gave up their function, and how now she was dependent on hemodialysis. She added how problematic was the insertion of her central venous line, and how desperately she depended on this plastic tube. (The placement of a central venous line in an individual with such severe scoliosis and contortion of the spine is very difficult.) I sensed that now, after the first month of hemodialysis with all its accompanying difficulties, she was starting to realize that it was not a temporary thing, but a permanent treatment with a huge impact on her life.

While we were talking about the impact of this new treatment, she gradually calmed down. Her movements became slower and more coordinated, and she seemed to go back to her usual even mood. In that session I got the feeling that the art-making process helped her to open up and to release verbally what was bothering her. She seemed to be able to contain herself by understanding what was going on within her.

The next session she produced several pencil drawings of "abstract figures." While up to this point her drawings were almost monochromatic, during this session she started to use color in a different, more playful way by filling in shapes. She seemed to enjoy exploring the matching of colors. That day she worked quietly, in an even way, totally absorbed in what she was doing. She did not want to make any comments nor associations about her piece of art. Unfortunately, we had to stop earlier than planned because, as a result of her being in a sitting position, her line started to have difficulties. I was surprised how easily she took this setback.

In the sixth session I had to remind her that the program was coming to an end. She decided to start something totally new, and together we went through the available possibilities. After a while she decided to work with pipe cleaners and feathers, even though she didn't know how to use them. So I showed her an example: by bending and twisting pipe cleaners I made her a simple butterfly. She was fascinated by this technique and immediately made an abstract shape, very similar to the ones she had been drawing during the previous session. When she was done, she asked me to make a girl for her, then indicated the exact colors and gesture of the body. Satisfied with this product, she made another abstract figure. For the rest of the time, we worked together on a joint project, her making abstract shapes, and I fulfilling what she was asking for. At the end of the session she had a final, satisfied look at the seven items we produced, and wanted to know what we were going to do with them. After a brief brainstorming session, she came up with the idea of a mobile, and asked me to bring some sticks to the next session (Figure 3.6: Untitled, mobile by Joan, 17 years).

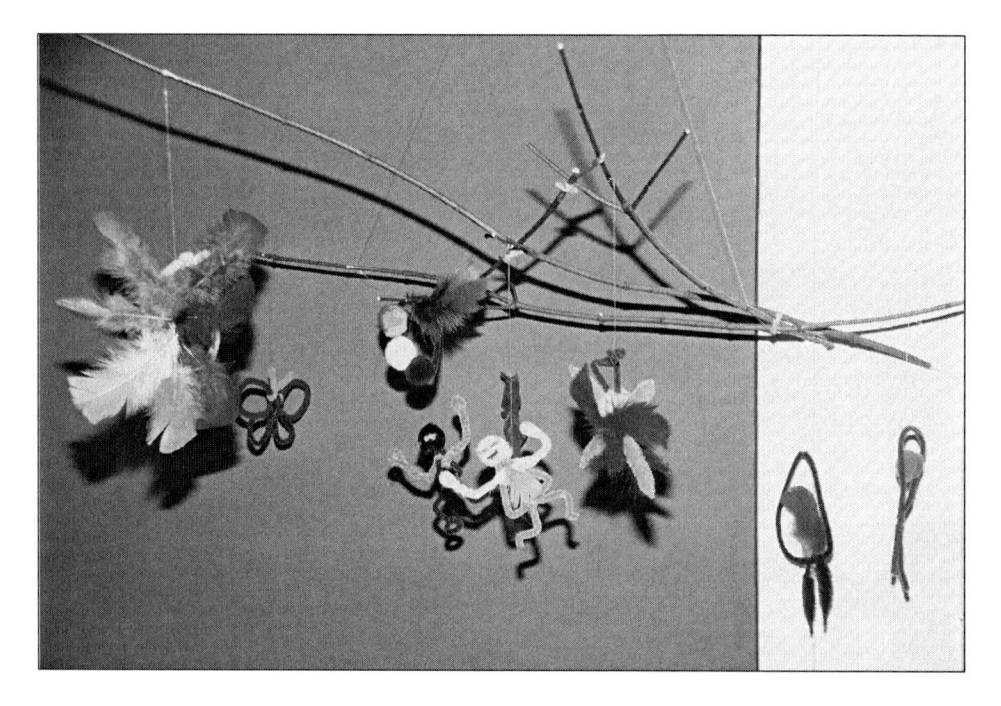

Figure 3.6. Untitled, mobile by Joan, 17 years.

During the following session she gave me as precise directions as possible as to how I had to tie together the tree branches, helping me as much as she could. The arrangement of the free-floating items took up the rest of the session. She carefully planned where each item had to hang, considering and evaluating possible interactions. After a final, satisfied look she decided to take it home right away. As if she wanted to exercise and explore her newly achieved creative skills, she decided to make a similar mobile in the remaining sessions, only this time working on her own, only asking for help when there was no other option. It was as if these free-floating objects were opening the horizon of her own restricted mobility, and were offering her a new dimension of freedom.

Although I was told about her developmental delay – that of having the level of a nine-year-old – I found it very difficult to evaluate her. She showed remarkable discrepancies in the different areas of development. I do not have the ability to assess her intellectual skills. However, the way her immediate action (content of drawing) was always linked to the content of her conversation lead to the assumption that she had not yet developed the capability of abstract thinking. Her cognitive development was still in the concrete stage of a nine- to ten-year-old. Considering her emotional development, she definitely showed much more advanced maturity. Her strength was her readiness to take risks, to head in new directions, trying new things without fearing failure. In case of a disappointment she showed a mature impulse control and good resilience in developing problem-solving strategies; and if she needed help she was able to ask for it in a very natural and appropriate way.

The most striking thing was her body perception. Her figure drawings and her clay figures reflected the body image of a three- to four-year-old child. Two things did not really match this developmental stage: the lack of her use of colors and the lack of orientation on a sheet of paper (ungrounded figures and objects). I began wondering if that was part of her severely disturbed body image, or was the result of the crooked growth of her own body and, therefore, distorted orientation in space. Her emotional stability with her characteristic way of positive thinking did not at all fit with the colorless, ungrounded and chaotic pictures. However, when she started to elaborate on the idea of a mobile with a free-floating quality, I had the feeling she was trying to overcome her immense physical restriction and to extend her horizon by exploring a new dimension of freedom.

SUMMARY

Seventeen-year-old Joan was very well able to connect with me. Due to her severe congenital impairment she had to deal with huge physical restrictions. Her bodily and facial malformation often were the reasons for being left out and avoided by other people. Nevertheless she seemed to have developed a fairly strong personality thanks to her very supportive close and extended family. For the whole time we spent together she was involved in her artwork. Her strength was her readiness to try things out without fearing failure, just enjoying the simple fact that somebody beside her family members spent time with her and paid her attention. Often I had the feeling she was using me as a tool, an extended arm or additional hand to overcome her physical restriction. Her art often was an attempt to extend her limited horizon.

3. Martin, Male, 15 Years

Description of the Client

Martin is a blond, 15-year-old Caucasian boy. He is of average size for his age and shows strong body features. His pubertal development is well advanced.

From the very beginning Martin was shy and withdrawn, and appeared easily embarrassed. His interaction with me was polite, but always careful; he kept me at a safe distance. He rarely talked spontaneously, but readily answered my questions in a friendly, but somehow uninvolved way, as if he was telling me about somebody else. Friendly avoidance was his typical behavior.

Social History

At the time, Martin was an average student in grade 10. He preferred spending his life fishing and adventuring in nature on his own rather than sitting at a school desk. He is the middle of three children and had an eighteen-year-old brother and a thirteen-year-old sister. His mother is a housewife, his father an employee in a construction tools store. Both parents are very engaged and supportive caregivers to their children. The family owned their own house. The most important person for Martin apart from members of his immediate family is his maternal grandmother. At times she seemed even closer to Martin than his mother. Apparently Martin did not have a lot of friends with which he could spend time, though he did have two very close friends who shared his love for withdrawal into nature.

Medical History

Martin was born with only one dysplastic kidney, which was working well until some years ago. Gradually this single kidney had given up its function over the previous few months, giving the family enough time to ready everybody for the transplantation. The extended testing for compatibility showed his brother to be the ideal organ donor. The well-functioning family prepared for the event very carefully, even developing an observer's role for the sister. The fact that Martin's brother is artistically highly skilled gave the parents the idea to ask for art therapy support for Martin during the whole procedure.

Art Therapy Process and Artwork

When I met Martin for the first time, he received his second hemodialysis in preparation for the transplant. Patiently, but displaying little interest, he followed the introduction and demonstration of the available art material. Immediately he let me know that he was not really into art, like his brother; and that maybe it was worth to invest in his brother rather than in him. I immediately sensed a mix of anger and surrender. First I reassured him that it was he I was interested in. As a second step we again went through the meaning of the art in this therapeutic approach. I stressed that it would all be confidential and that the emphasis was on using the material to express positive and negative feelings rather than to make nice art. I confirmed to him that the expression "art" in this therapeutic approach was misleading, because it suggested having artistic skills, and knowledge about aesthetics; and that what we were doing here was quite different from what his brother was doing on canvas. He agreed to give art therapy a trial and finished the session by writing his name in colorful letters onto the cover of his folder.

Three days later he got his surgical intervention. Everything went well. For the next two weeks I visited him a few times. Due to pain he was not able to sit and make art. As a result, we spent the next session just talking and making plans for future projects. It was then when he told me about his hobbies and sporting activities, like hockey and baseball. When he was not at school or hanging around outdoors in nature, he liked to construct small plastic models, following precise construction plans and instructions for the painting. He seemed to double-check with me if that was also the kind of art I was talking about. I assured him that this could be a starting point for the two of us. At the end of the session his mother reminded him to show me the photographs of his brother's most recent painting in all its stages of creation, which was obviously the family's pride. Since Martin apparently was part of the project, and hoping to get further information about my client, I agreed to have a look at them. The picture was a huge acrylic painting about Martin's brother's life, including the recent surgical intervention in graffiti style. Not only was the depiction of the operation that the two brothers shared part of the painting, Martin was also allowed to paint some sections. I could sense some pride when Martin showed me the small areas of the farthest background he was allowed to paint. "It is about his life, and I am a small part of it," as Martin explained his brother's painting to me. But where Martin saw accomplishment, I had the impression of the subordinate, admiring behavior of one of Da Vinci's disciples, who was allowed to paint the background of a cloud. Was that the confirmation for what I had assumed? Did Martin spent most of his life in the shadow of his brilliant older brother, who seemed to be very independent, brave and successful, and an excellent artist on top? Both parents seemed to love all their children, but their favorite – no doubt – was their oldest son; and their most needy child was Martin. After I got this additional information about the family dynamics, I started to wonder about what kind of effect the previous surgery had on Martin. The opposite to what Musial (1984) described in her chapter seemed to happen in this family. In most families the living related kidney donor seemed to be neglected, and lacked appreciation for what he/she did. In this family Martin's brother appeared to be the generous hero who took the risk of a sacrifice to save his brother's life, whereas Martin was pushed into an even more dependent and subordinate position regarding his brother. Compared to his brother he was always weaker; even his body never worked well. He had to be happy and grateful to have his brother saving his life. One could imagine what kind of influence that could have on Martin's self-esteem. I started to understand why he tried to hide behind his brother's back, and regress to the position of the family's baby.

I decided to cut off the theme of the gifted brother and to concentrate on Martin's needs. So for the next session I suggested to Martin that he bring his plastic models in order to show me what he is interested in, and maybe to teach me some new techniques. I was hoping to show him how important he was to me. Somehow it was difficult for me to tolerate his emotional pain.

As we had established for the third session, Martin brought in his models. I was very surprised to learn that his favorite theme was war, including soldiers, tanks and war planes. Was that the way this quiet, withdrawn, adolescent boy vented his hidden anger and frustration related to sibling rivalry? Never before had he been so talkative with me as he explained all the technical features of these machines and the differences between the soldier's uniforms and how, at home, he had a whole collection of soldiers of all parties of the Second World War and of the Vietnam War. For a while I listened to his enthusiastic narration in order to give him the attention he desperately needed. Then I tried carefully to switch the theme to a more technical aspect, asking questions about the work process and special material he was using. Hoping to move towards a more spontaneous creative process (leaving detailed construction maps) I suggested that we could make a landscape for his models next time.

When I met him for the next session he was tired but in a good mood. He announced that he had become an outpatient due to his unexpectedly fast recovery after surgery, and that he was living with his beloved grandmother because he still had to show up at the hospital on a daily basis. When I asked him about today's plan for the session, he replied that he had his father take home all his models because he had to move to his grandmother's place. After a while he decided to make a quick drawing. I had the feeling it was less triggered by his own urge, but represented more an attempt to please me and to connect with me. Since he loved nature, I suggested a tree drawing, giving him the appropriate assignments, to bridge his lack of ideas (Figure 3.7: "My Tree," drawing by Martin, 15 years). (Assignments according to Bolander (1977): Draw a tree representing you, focusing on season, environment, weather conditions, etc.).

He agreed to make this quick drawing for me, refusing to use colors. Obviously he was not interested in investing too much in this drawing. Beside the given information about the season (winter), he did not want to process the picture further. But I did wonder about the four flowers blooming in wintertime that he drew, while his tree had no leaves. Did they symbolize the healthy rest of his family? Other striking features were the missing ground, the overall sad mood and lifelessness, despite the blooming flowers. Was that just the mirror of his lack of engagement? Or was there a hint of depressed mood? According to Bolander (1977) the three parts of a tree (roots, trunk and crown) represent the three spheres (instinctual nature, emotional life and spiritual development). However, due to the lack of engagement shown by Martin, I was hesitant to make interpretations. Nevertheless I wondered about the metaphoric message of this tree. Its crown dominated by the number three showed a striking mixture of hanging branches and fork-shaped pointed main branches. I got a sense of anger and aggression combined with sadness, which was reinforced by the lifelessness of this empty winter landscape.

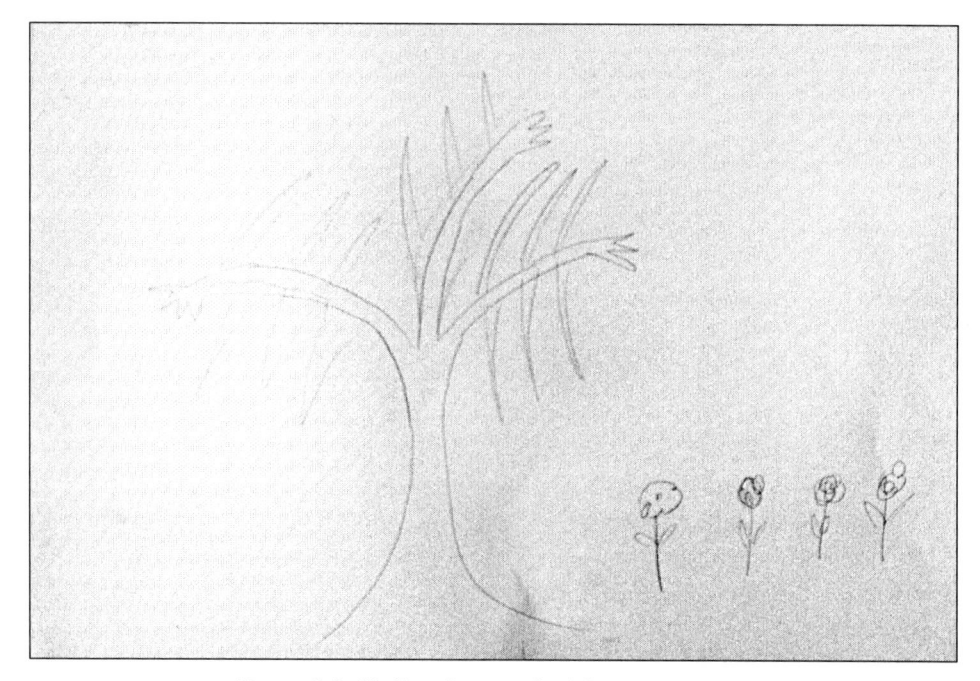

Figure 3.7. *My Tree*, drawing by Martin, 15 years.

His models didn't make it for our next session either. They were at home now, he said, where he'd gone to a month earlier, leaving his grandmother's house (the plan was that he'd come to the hospital on a weekly basis for bloodwork). Instead, Martin asked for a directive and he decided to draw a picture, again more to please me than for his own need. Choosing a simple pencil, he followed the assignment of the bridge drawing (Figure 3.8: "A Bridge," drawing by Martin, 15 years). (Hays (1981), Assignment: "Draw a bridge focusing on construction, obstacle to overcome (e.g., river, canyon, etc.), environment and traffic direction crossing the bridge, indicating in a second step with a mark where you would stand in relation to the bridge, and in which direction you are heading.")

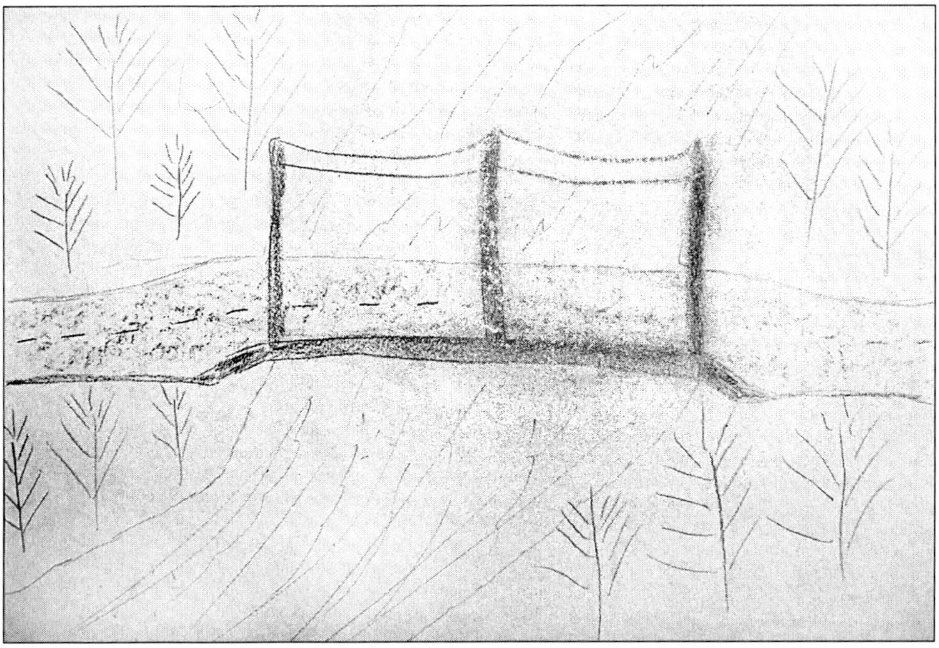

Figure 3.8. *A Bridge*, drawing by Martin, 15 years.

This time Martin was more into what he was doing, and the result was definitely richer. He told me about the big, fast flowing river under the bridge leading a lot of water, about the dense forest on either end of the bridge where one could get lost, and about the two lanes of the bridge allowing traffic in both directions. He stressed the importance of the high railing of the bridge in order to protect people from falling down because the river was dangerous. Finally, he told me he would stand on the middle of the bridge, "maybe a little further to the right side, heading to the right." But he did not want to make a mark where he would see himself standing. My question about the safety of the bridge he answered with "It's pretty stable." For all the danger surrounding it, to me this bridge appeared fragile and only loosely fixed at the shore of the river. Its high banister left several dangerous spots (on either end and underneath) from which one could fall into the river. To me this picture perhaps was a metaphoric expression of Martin's vulnerability and insecurity, and for his need for support, attention and protection.

When I met him for the sixth session – and, I learned the week later by his mother, the last one – he was tired, and he did not feel like doing anything. He told me about the renovation work on his house and how he would work on his soldier models on a regular basis. With pride he told me how he discovered a new field of interest: all kinds of vehicles, focusing mainly on trucks and planes, not for wars but for public use. I was surprised, and suspicious, doubting that he was able to leave his anger behind him and to move on after only a few weeks of treatment. Did he sense my difficulties in tolerating his anger, and therefore, told me this to please me?

A week later he let me know through his mother that he wanted to quit art therapy because he did not want to spend extra time at the hospital. However, he did want to leave me his drawings as a souvenir. A last attempt to connect with me? Or a last sign for his need for attention? I wondered about the real reason for this unexpected dropping out. Did he feel threatened by the power of expression through art after his two drawing sessions? Did he try to avoid any kind of artistic expression, as a sign of opposition and rebellion against his brother's power?

SUMMARY

Fifteen-year-old Martin was reluctant to join the art therapy program, and finally dropped out. In his withdrawn and shy manner, he seemed to hide behind the back of his artistically very talented brother, kidney donor and pride of the family. He suffered of a weak self-esteem. With the exception of the two pencil drawing Martin refused to use the offered art material, but preferred to work with his model soldiers and weapons. To me his artwork was the metaphor for his unconscious anger and aggression he could not release in another way. Unfortunately, he was not hospitalized long enough to develop a trustful working alliance between the two of us. Maybe art therapy was not the ideal approach for Martin, representing the detested means of expression of his brilliant brother. Maybe the risk of comparison between the two brothers was too high and too humiliating for Martin.

B. LONG-TERM TREATMENT GROUP

4. Abdul, Male, 16 Years

Description of the Client

Abdul is a tall, slim, sixteen-year-old teenager of Indian origin. With his dark skin and smooth black hair he has an attractive appearance. His even movements underline his calm character. He was naturally open and had a friendly way of encountering people, a politeness often observed in Indian culture.

Abdul is bright with excellent academic skills, despite interruptions from school due to his illness. He has a healthy curiosity and likes to spend time engaged in research and self-education. His dream is to become a lawyer. He is more a thinker than a talker, but likes to share experiences and discoveries, and have discussions with people he trusts. He is warm and engaging and makes quick eye contact. He is capable of good back-and-forth communication, and retains a good, healthy sense of humor.

At the start, he was excessively polite, like that of a real gentleman. Over time, Abdul became demanding and manipulative, demonstrating defiant-rejective behavior. But after even more time, he showed a mature, interactive behavior on an equal level as peers. Throughout, he exhibited a well-developed creativity and age-appropriate abstract thinking.

His mood was even. He had good impulse control, and never showed anger. He was more of a passive-aggressive type of personality, showing avoidance when angry. In general he tried to hide his emotions and not lose face. He seemed to know his limitations and tended not to push or go beyond them in order to avoid the need for help.

His positive thinking fueled his explorative behavior, and he increasingly developed the strength to take risks. His initial response of suspicion and withdrawal to my questions about an actual piece of art changed with time into a hesitant attempt to explore the depth of his art.

One of Abdul's strengths was his absolute reliability and his strict, almost compulsive compliance. He was often called the "exemplary patient." Another strength was his good sense of humor and, related to that, his optimism: he would try to push further a good quality, instead of despairing for a bad one. I never saw him give up.

Social History

Two years before the two of us met, Abdul's parents and their two children left India for North America to join relatives. By immigrating the parents hoped to offer their children a better education and better opportunities for a good job, perhaps even an academic education at a university. But two weeks after the family arrived, Abdul became severely sick.

Abdul's parents appeared intelligent and genuinely interested in what was good for their son. The family's religious background is Hindu, although they did not practice the faith. The father had been married previously, but had lost his first wife to disease. He has six adult children from his first marriage; they had remained in India. Abdul's mother, the father's second wife, was ten years younger and gave birth to two children: Abdul's sister, 18 years of age, and Abdul, 16 years. Before they left India the family lived in New Delhi, where both parents worked as government employees in areas of taxation and accountancy. Thanks to the parents' high government positions, both children went through an English-speaking school system and grew up bilingual with Hindi. Following tradition, they lived close to their extended family, especially on the paternal side. The maternal side of the family had left India for North America in 1985. On emigrating the parents had to give up their high positions and good jobs in India. Now they were both working at the airport, in jobs supplying food for airlines. They both had the feeling that they were starting from zero because their qualifications were not recognized here. But both were willing to make these sacrifices for the sake of their offspring. Whereas the mother missed India and dreamed of returning one day, the father was trying to adjust to life here as quickly as possible.

After her arrival, Abdul's sister started her education in the field of human resources and was able to get a job. The siblings apparently had a very close relationship. The whole family system seemed to be very supportive of Abdul and, at the same time, was well embedded in an extended family of maternal aunts and cousins.

Abdul had only a few good friends who shared his interests. He had no girlfriend. In general, he seemed to be rather selective in his friendships. Abdul's pride, which often made it necessary for him to hide his emotions, sometimes acted as a social barrier as well. He often felt too superior and too educated to get involved with certain people, which made contacts with peers difficult.

Medical History

Abdul was a wanted child. Pregnancy and delivery were normal. He was always a strong, healthy child with normal developmental milestones. He was never severely ill, nor had he had surgery. According to his mother, he was always an "easy child," very calm, judicious and ambitious.

Two weeks after Abdul's arrival he became severely sick, with vomiting and near-loss of consciousness, and had to be hospitalized. At the Intensive Care Unit (ICU) doctors found an end-stage renal failure of unknown origin. Despite all their testing they couldn't find a cause for this failure, though they did suspect the problem had been building for some time. It had nothing, they believed, to do with immigration. The parents maintained otherwise. However, at the hospital all the people involved in the case knew why the family had to keep this stance: If you mention a preexisting physical or mental defect to immigration officials, you will never get the authorization to immigrate – you will be sent back immediately. But if you acquire a disease after immigration, they have to keep you.

At the hospital, Abdul needed to be put on hemodialysis immediately. During the next months of hemodialysis, high blood pressure was always an issue and, as a result, he was heavily medicated. Two months prior to our meeting, Abdul had a so-called "hypertensive crisis," a state in which blood pressure becomes almost uncontrollably high despite compliance in taking medication. In these cases, the risk for cerebral hemorrhages is extremely high. The only way to get the situation under control was the immediate removal of both of Abdul's kidneys. As a consequence, by the time I met him he was definitively dependent on regular and intensive hemodialysis.

During the art therapy program Abdul went through a highly sophisticated testing for transplant, a procedure which usually takes two months of ongoing tests and examinations. Much to everyone's puzzlement, including my own, he absolutely refused to have his family tested even though he knew that living-donor transplantation through family would have a much better outcome. Although he was told that he would probably have to wait two to three years for a cadaver-kidney because of his very rare blood group, he maintained his rigid position.

Abdul was lucky. On a weekend half-way through the art therapy program, he was transplanted with a kidney that suddenly became available. It was a big event for all participants! Due to his compliance and positive thinking, Abdul recovered quickly and the kidney functioned perfectly.

Art Therapy Process and Artwork

We started the art therapy program, which lasted 34 sessions. By reviewing Abdul's art I realized that our work went through four main stages, each with its peculiar interactions, transference and countertransference.

The *first stage* of forming a trustful working alliance by going through a lot of resistance lasted for about eight weeks. After the introduction and demonstration of the available art material, Abdul decided to start by decorating the cover of his folder with watercolor (Figure 3.9: Untitled, watercolor by Abdul, 16 years).

He spent two sessions working on this picture. While painting the sun and the multilayered profile of a human face, he told me he wanted to make the same picture he had made when he had been in grade six back home in India. He got an award for that, but he had to leave it behind when they left. He then told me about his two favorite teachers in India, both art teachers. One was a great artist who was able to paint light in a magnificent way. Both were Abdul's role models, although he also maintained that he would like to become a lawyer, not an artist. Another theme was his family, especially his paternal half-siblings, who remained in India with their families, and how much he missed them. While he started to paint a bright blue sky, he told me about India and how the country would now be experiencing the end of Monsoon rain. "I was born in August and I brought a lot of water with me" was his comment. But then he decided to add two trees in spring. Obviously, he was missing India, still having very strong roots there, whereas he had not really been able to put down roots here yet.

While finishing his painting at the next session, he told me about school: He was in grade eleven and tried to keep up, although he had to miss many classes. He told me about his spare time and how he liked to hang around with friends and go to the movies. Later, I learned through his social worker that he had big troubles at school because of his frequent absences every Monday, Wednesday and Friday. His life took place at home, at the hospital and in-between on the subway, one way taking him one and a half hours. Three hours of subway trip added to the four hours of dialysis three times a week certainly did not give him much spare time.

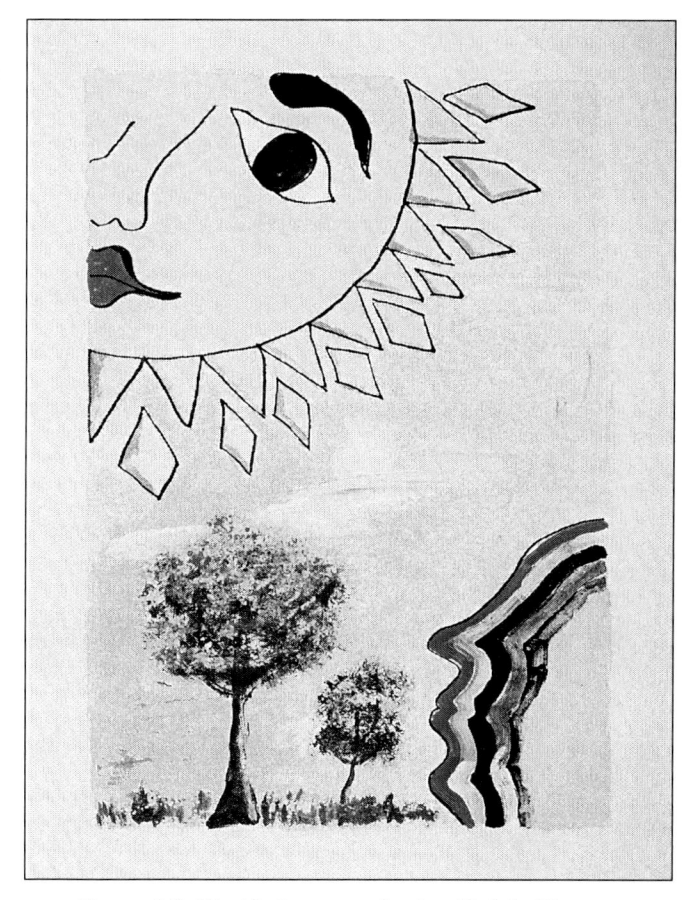

Figure 3.9. Untitled, watercolor by Abdul, 16 years.

Throughout these first two art therapy sessions he planned his picture carefully, using pencil and eraser before coloring with paint. I perceived his meticulousness about aesthetics to be not just part of his Indian heritage, but that it was also a nice curtain to hide behind. At the same time, he tried hard to connect with me and to please me. However, he did not want to talk further about this first picture.

For the next session he decided to make another watercolor painting, but without using pencil and eraser (Plate 1: "A Landscape," watercolor by Abdul, 16 years, p. 45).

It was while painting this landscape that he told me for the first time about his problems at school – and that he had dropped out. Now, he was starting at a so-called credit school, where it did not matter how many hours one spent in class. Instead, one completed assignments in order to get credits.

This time he was a bit more willing to talk about the picture when he was done. So I asked him about the mountains. He told me that there were no mountains where he was coming from, and that he hated mountains and loved flat landscapes. The associations he gave me to this piece of art was about the flooding river, which occurred every year in August in his country; that was the month when he was born. (It was October when he created the picture.)

According to Oster and Gould (1987) the use of the space of a sheet of paper may give important information about the perception of an individual's lifespan e.g., whereas the right half of an image may reveal information about the individuals perception of future, the left half is more related to the past.

Although the right side of the picture appeared to be unfinished, Abdul was done with the painting. I thought the huge river flowing to the left side (back to the past) was about India and the flooding after the Monsoon rain, the period when he left his country. I perceived the mountains to be insuperable barriers: again a wall to hide behind. The striking thing was the emptiness of the right half of the paper (related to the future). Obviously, he had no perception of his presence there. And there was no bridge or boat or anything else that could be used to cross the river and connect both shores. Despite the rich vegetation, there was no other sign of life other than two trees, both standing at the right-hand side of the river. I thought they might have represented less the two countries, and perhaps more the two of us, still keeping a secure distance. I also wondered if the sunset over the river was a metaphor for his mourning for the loss of his country.

During this session the alarm of his machine went off repeatedly. I was surprised by his autonomy and his ability to press buttons and regulate his blood flow. Each time he informed the nurse about the changes he performed, explaining to me: "I'm having control, but telling them what I changed means not having the responsibility for what I did."

The next session was the first day at his credit school and for a while I observed him with the teacher who came to the hospital to work with him. He seemed to have fun. We started art therapy after his school, and he was in an excellent mood.

First he looked at his cover for a long time, obviously with pleasure. "I especially like the figure, maybe because it could be me," he said. I tried to find out more, but he quickly changed the subject, asked for a new piece of paper and watercolor, and for a directive. So I asked him for a bridge drawing, giving him the recommended assignment (Hays, 1981) (Plate 2: "A Day of Celebration," watercolor by Abdul, 16 years, p. 45).

When he was done with the bridge drawing he made me guess where the bridge was leading, adding that the traffic was going from the left to the right. He was very pleased with my correct guess. While adding the fireworks in the sky, he titled the picture "A Day of Celebration." When I asked him about where he would be in relation to the bridge, he added two black figures holding hands onto the left river shore. "Father and son watching the fireworks together" was his answer.

Although the bridge was very stable and made of stone, there were no railings. I was concerned about safety, and wondered about the city at the end of the bridge, which seemed to be so far away and almost unreachable, like a very light and distant dream. Without having a concrete idea about the beginning of the bridge, and acknowledging the two figures on the "past side" of the river, I wondered if and how Abdul would be able to reach the bridge, and if he was able to connect the old with the new world, his past with his future. I had the feeling he lacked a sense not only of the future, but also for the present. And suddenly, the bridge seemed to become more a barrier than a connection.

With Halloween coinciding with our fifth session I noticed a gradual change in behavior. Abdul seemed to be unusually distractible and irritable. His submissive, polite behavior changed into a more arrogant withdrawal. Suddenly he did not like my questions anymore and he tried to totally avoid the subject of his origin. Around the same time he switched to different art materials: oil pastels, pipe cleaners, clay, and so on (Plate 3: "The Green Step Towards the Sun," oil pastels, and "Running Man," pipe cleaners by Abdul, 16 years, p. 46).

The next piece was done in oil pastels. While he explained to me about the sun at the upper left corner and the Earth at the lower right, he quickly added four black profiles into the four corners. I had no doubt that the foot with only four toes represented himself, his now defective wholeness. When I asked him if green had a special meaning for him or his culture he reacted with annoyance, and refused to answer. At this point in time I did not comment on his oppositional behavior. I did later, though. His reaction was denial explaining to me that he "simply did not want to talk about his art and did not like all the stupid questions about it."

For the next two months he would show the same oppositional reaction to my questions. While playing with the pipe cleaners and making the "Running Man," he told me in a firm voice that he did not like his art teacher. Although he knew perfectly well that I was not an art teacher, I sensed his rejection, that he was trying to put me back to a safe distance. Was the "Running Man" the metaphor for his own attempt to run away? In his tenseness and irritability I could feel his ambivalence, his being pushed and pulled between two poles (e.g., the burning hot sun and the cool earth). I wondered if it was about the two cultures, or if it was the beginning struggle between him and his transferential me, or if it was the arising of adolescent issues now that he was finally able to let fall the facade of his politeness? Was he challenging authority? Or was he afraid of the power of the artwork, of sexual feelings in himself, or towards me? There was no way to address his change in demeanor; and therefore, we will never get an answer to all these questions.

At the next session he was high-spirited and highly distractible. He decided to make a watercolor painting (Figure 3.10: Untitled, watercolor by Abdul, 16 years).

While painting a red-haired woman, he did not talk to me spontaneously, nor did he make eye contact. I sensed his confusion while he was struggling with the facial features. He then covered everything with a nice pink color, leaving just the vibrant red lips spared. I could feel his embarrassment as he painted the contour of the breasts onto the purple sweater, which he then tried to hide by making up "crossed arms." I did not have to ask him if he knew this woman because, towards the end of the session, his social worker with her assistant, interrupted our session. Immediately, I knew that the painting was of her because of her red hair and excessive red lipstick. After the two women left us he added the background to the picture. Were all this turbulence and these colors representing his own inner agitation and turmoil about sexual attraction?

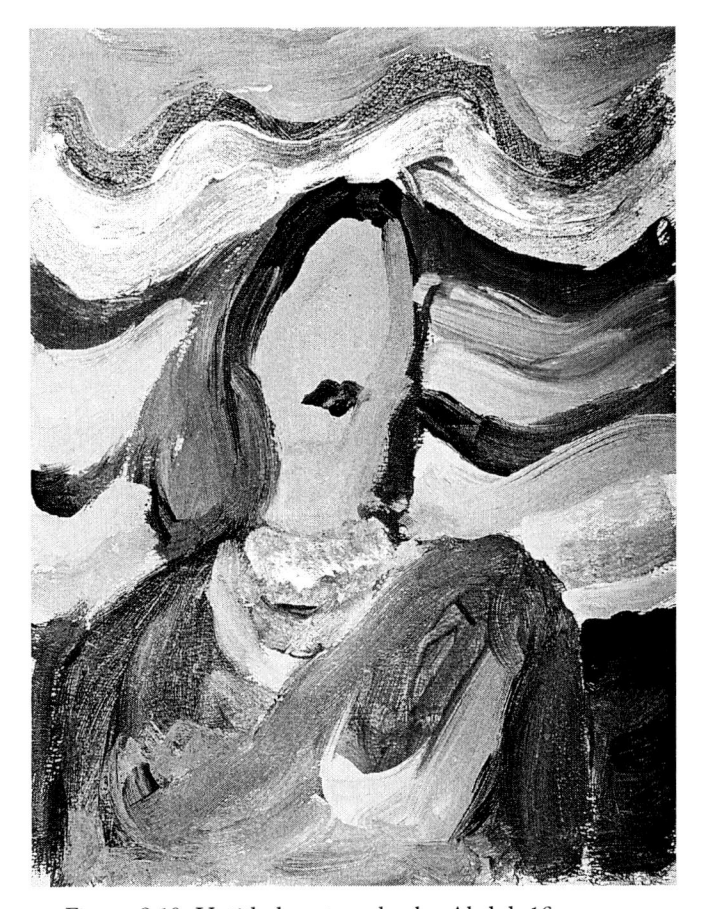

Figure 3.10. Untitled, watercolor by Abdul, 16 years.

With Halloween there was a big shift in his behavior. He started to be annoyed by my questions about his art, showing suspicion and concerns about my possible interpretations, as if fearing that interpretations of his artworks represented some sort of control over him. More and more, he lost his polite behavior and, at the same time, his aesthetic control over his pictures. I could sense his ambivalence between attraction and rejection, between engagement and withdrawal, between interactive communication and letting me down. I felt his defiance growing, maybe caused by a discomfort that he felt concerning the loss of control over his art.

The *second stage*, during which Abdul showed a behavior of provocation and testing boundaries, lasted for about twelve weeks.

At the next session he wanted to work in charcoal, a technique new to him. For that purpose he wanted to have a photograph that he could copy. Flipping through my collage material he found a face of a young man (Figure 3.11: Untitled, charcoal by Abdul, 16 years).

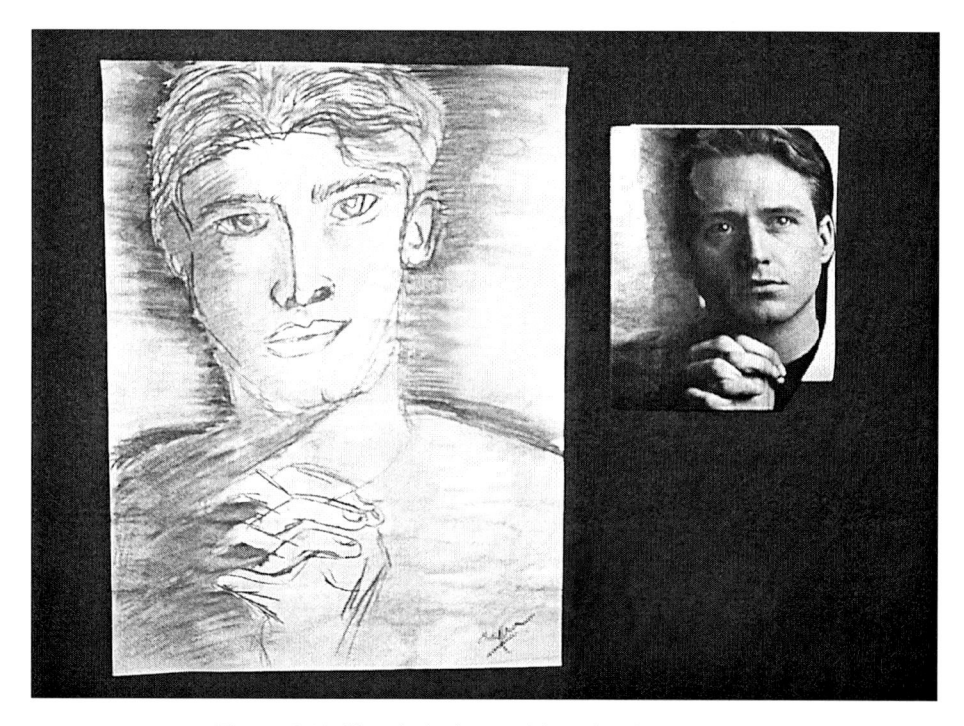

Figure 3.11. Untitled, charcoal by Abdul, 16 years.

While he was working, he told me about a self-portrait he had to make at school and how difficult the assignment was. "Because you cannot draw you nicer than you really are. In fact, you are just who you are," was his comment.

For the next several weeks he stuck with the same technique, asking for more photographs of faces, but only young, nice faces. Whatever photographs I brought, he found something in them to be critical of – either the face was not young enough, or it was too ugly. Finally, I started to understand that the whole discussion about the models in the photographs perhaps reflected the power control issue between the two of us. He was asking for support for his drawings, but he would also blame me afterwards for controlling his artistic activities. As a result, I suggested that from now he would be responsible for bringing in his own photographs of models from magazines collected over the week. But he never did.

Gradually Abdul's behavior towards me became more and more defiant and rejective. At the same time, he showed a sweet, flirtatious behavior with the nurses. By aligning himself with them, he definitely seemed to be trying to make me feel like an outsider or intruder. During the session he withdrew, spoke little and made no eye contact. When he did talk, there was a strong undertone of annoyance and impatience in his voice. He presented the typical signs of passive aggression and showed a very demanding and manipulative behavior towards me. Was he fighting against his transferential me of authority, parental figure, doctor or other control figure representing the hospital? Or was he defensive against sexual feelings towards me (erotic transference)? This behavior would match with his developmental stage of an adolescent.

After about eight weeks of defiance, his behavior started to change gradually again. At this session he asked for chalk pastels, though he continued to stick with photographic models (Plate 4: Untitled, chalk pastels by Abdul, 16 years, p. 46).

Although chalk pastels apparently were new to him, he showed amazing ability with them. During this session Abdul was friendlier, made good eye contact and was very talkative. He told me about the wedding of one of his cousins back home, and how expensive those marvelous Indian wedding dresses were because they were all hand-made of silk. He seemed to be back to his good mood again.

For the next four weeks not only did his behavior turn into a more mature interaction with me, he also became more willing to expand on his themes. So instead of looking for photographs of people, now he also wanted shots of landscapes and houses for his more colorful work in chalk pastels.

At one session, after having chosen chalk pastels, he switched to pencil (Figure 3.12: Untitled, pencil drawing by Abdul, 16 years).

He chose the face of a middle-aged, African American businessman. While telling me about his new fascination with archaeology and the evolution of humans, he started to change the face step-by-step and to make his own interpretation. He even added hands with weapons. He obviously was enjoying this process – and was very surprised about the unplanned way in which he changed the man's face.

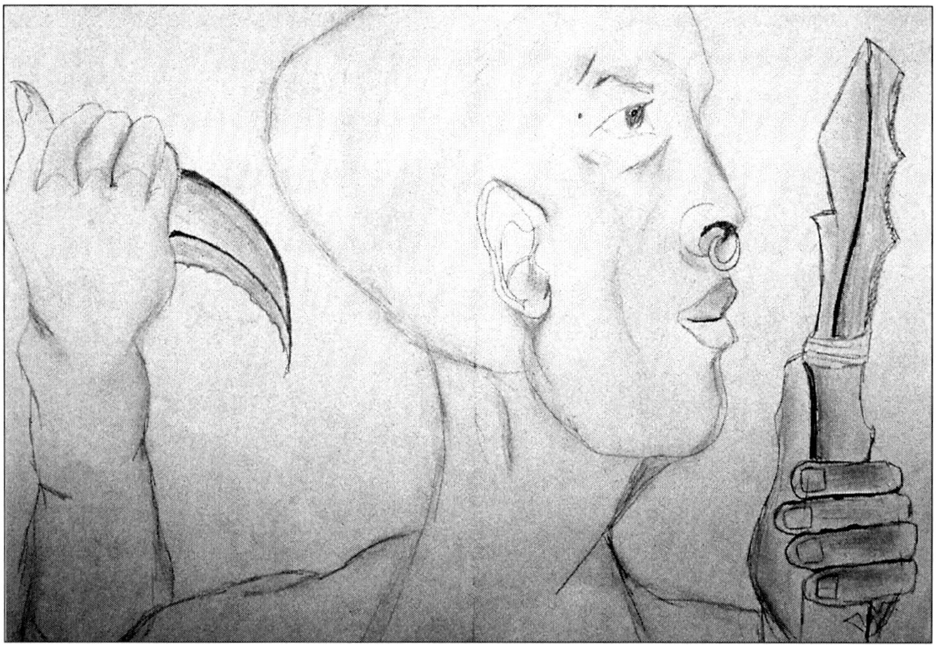

Figure 3.12. Untitled, pencil drawing by Abdul, 16 years.

Again we had a good time – and an intense conversation. For a while we talked about the importance of making one's own interpretations rather than just copying what other artists and photographers had already done. We were celebrating the fact that he had made his first interpretation of a picture, one that showed that he was developing some autonomy in terms of having an opinion and point of view about something.

At the next session Abdul started to tell me about the visit of his cousins from Florida, and that he would be their guide in the city. It was a nice opportunity for him to explore and discover his environment. I asked him if he had been in Florida himself. This question triggered a long conversation about the limitations of hemodialysis, the freedom transplantation would bring, and finally his hope that he would get a kidney some day, although he most likely would have to wait for a long time since he had a very rare blood type. I asked him if his family had been tested as potential donors, although I already knew the answer. He explained the reasons for his decision not to have them tested. First: he did not want to make them sick or incomplete like him, because one per family was enough; besides, he was now used to this kind of life. Second: he had been told that a transplanted organ would survive only ten to fifteen years, and therefore he would have to have several transplants during his life, but his family members could donate only one kidney, so he would always depend on kidneys from strangers. I sensed that these reasons were rationalizations as defense mechanism for deeper, unconscious conflicts. But at that time, I didn't know more than that.

While he was telling me these things, he was drawing another portrait (Figure 3.13: Untitled, pencil drawing by Abdul, 16 years.) This time, however, he put back the photograph of the African American man after a short time, deciding that he wanted to make his own interpretation of the person. This new, very masculine man looked much older and showed a certain superior self-confidence. I was surprised to find in this picture Abdul's own new facial features – a small beard on the chin, for example, and an extended growth of hair on the cheeks.

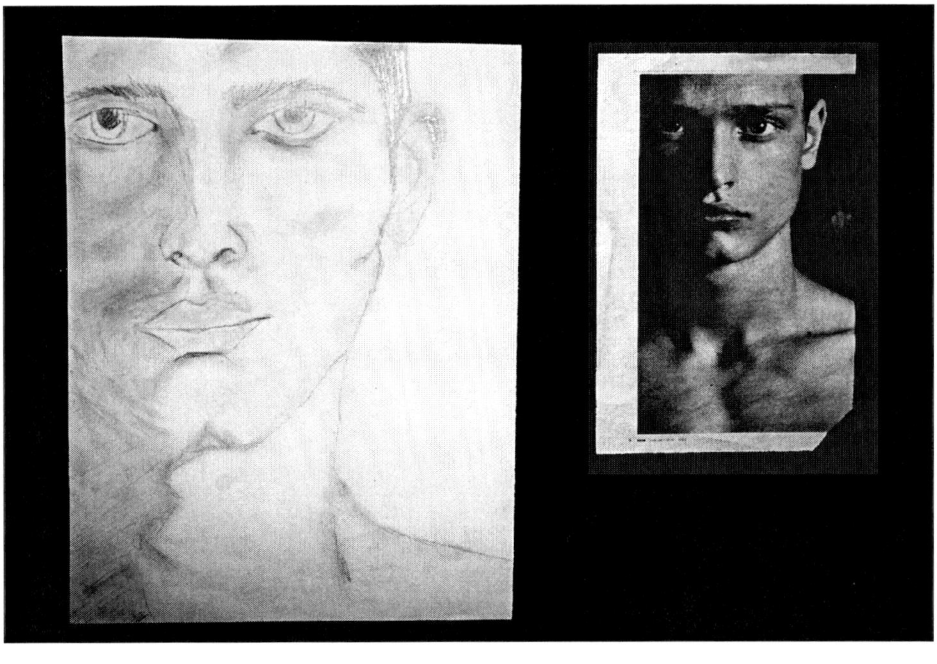

Figure 3.13. Untitled, pencil drawing by Abdul, 16 years.

Obviously Abdul was surprised by this new interpretation as well, what triggered the question about the definition of "good art" in him. That was a good and very difficult question. I remembered my own struggle at the school of art. I asked him how he would define "good art." Being a good artist to him meant knowing how to use material, being able to draw things as precisely and realistically as possible and being able to create aesthetic things. Apparently the addition of the artist's own interpretation of a reproduced piece was not part of Abdul's definition. The theme about aesthetics obviously was coming up on a more conscious level. I asked him why aesthetics were so important. Because people had to like what an artist was doing, he answered. "And what about the artist?" I asked. "He should like it as well," was his brief answer. "But the reality is that one cannot please everybody, so who is the most important person in this game?" was my question. He did not give me an answer, but I could see that he was honestly thinking about one.

The *third stage* lasted about two weeks and was triggered by the unexpected kidney transplantation.

When I visited Abdul as an inpatient 48 hours after his surgery, the nurses were trying to mobilize him for the first time. He wanted to see me immediately, telling the nurses that I was his therapist and he needed to see me. When I met him he was sitting, trembling and shaking in a hospital nightgown on a chair. I did not want to put him into the embarrassing situation where he would be seen by his female therapist in these loosely-dressed conditions. However, he obviously was not afraid of losing face and did not care about his appearance, but was happy to see me. Obviously he was under some sort of emotional shock and needed to talk. Over and over again he told me what had happened to him during the previous 48 hours. He talked of how totally unexpected was the 5 a.m. call on Saturday that told him to come to the hospital; of how all the checks with the donor kidney matched; and of how "there was no escape anymore" from entering the OR, and so forth. I had the feeling he was trying desperately to connect with the reality, or perhaps resolve or work through the trauma of surgery by telling me the same story at least four times. When he then started to explain to me the immunosuppression to avoid rejection of the kidney and the function of his morphine pump, with which he would control his pain by himself, I knew that he was back to reality again. When I left I had to promise to come back soon.

The next visit I met Abdul's mother, who would share his room for the duration of the two weeks he was an inpatient. Abdul was still in too much pain for making art. He told me that the doctors were encouraging him to leave the bed more often – and I could sense a non-verbalized "but." Spontaneously, I suggested that the three of us go for a walk together. He was almost waiting for this offer, but decided that his mother should wait in his room for him.

While we were walking, he told me again, for the last time, his story. Then he moved on to tell me about the amount of fluid intake. Now, he had to drink four to five liters a day, whereas before he was restricted to one. He also now had to take about 15 pills a day on a pretty strict schedule.

In this state of absolute regression he had his mother with him day and night, and he seemed to appreciate that. He told me once that it was the first time in his life he would have had to sleep away from his family in a foreign country. At the same time, however, for his first getting up from bed and his first walk through the hospital he chose not to do these activities with his mother; rather, he seemed to prefer doing them with me. This led me to wonder again about his transference towards me. During his stage of defiance, his transference was definitively one of authority, parental figure, control instance. But now in this stage of regression, he had his mother very close with him, and his transference towards me might have been more one of a good friend, a buddy who would admire him for what he had gone through.

For the next session he was waiting for me and was well enough to make art. He asked for pencil and eraser and an idea. He was not ready for my first suggestion to make a drawing about his newly changed circumstances, but felt attracted by the suggestion of doing a tree drawing (including the recommended assignment by Boland (1977)). (Figure 3.14: "My Tree," pencil drawing by Abdul, 16 years.)

Asking for white chalk pastel to add snow, he explained that it was winter (a time of regeneration and recovery) in his picture. I asked him about the windmill, and he told me about these typical Indian windmills with wooden wings. They were, he said, one of the simplest means with which to produce electricity as energy. Was that the metaphor for him being re-energized for whatever life might bring him? Or more a sign for his need for energy? At the same time the wooden wings reminded me of the pumping wheel of the dialysis machine. Not being dependent on it anymore, he was allowed now to put it into the background.

He added a connecting road between his tree and the windmill. Finally he squeezed another tree in-between the two items. His own tree was positioned more to the left-hand side of the paper and, therefore, according to Boland (1977), symbolizing mother binding. But at the same time, the tree's crown was bent to the right, and may symbolize his father's support as well. Although the tree had solid roots, it had a strikingly splitted trunk. Since according to Boland (1977) the trunk represents emotionality, I wondered if this split trunk could express a certain ambivalence. At the same time it reminded me a grafted branch, maybe representing his transplanted kidney, which was not yet totally a part of himself. And what about the second tree he drew last? Could that represent me standing beside him on his path of life?

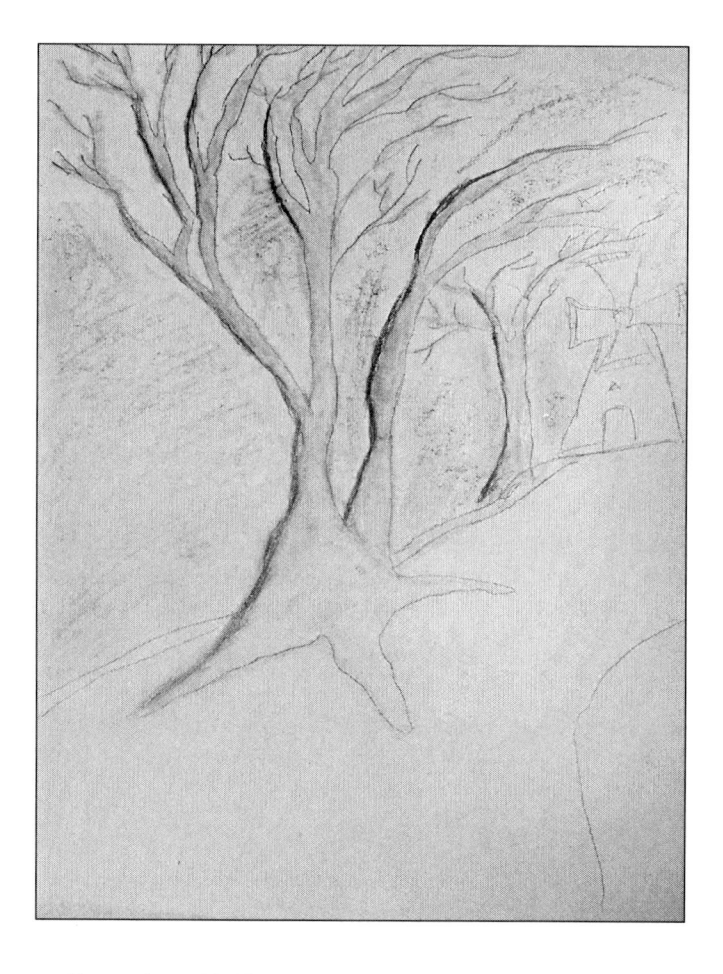

Figure 3.14. *My Tree*, pencil drawing by Abdul, 16 years.

The *fourth stage*, where Abdul was exploring the future, lasted for another twelve weeks.

Due to his positive thinking and his excellent compliance he recovered quickly from his surgery and was discharged after two weeks. As an outpatient he had initially to come for check-ups on a weekly basis; later, due to the increasing stability of his physical condition and good-working kidney, the doctors would increase the intervals between visits.

When I met Abdul for the first time after discharge he was nervous, and for the first time he allowed himself to show his feelings and to verbalize his anxiety with me. Although his kidney was working well and the control biopsy was perfect, he felt anxious because he had developed a heavy tremor in his hands due to the medication he was on. He chose an image of a male face and started to copy it with pencil, showing me through this regression that today he needed more containment due to the loss of control of his hands. He told me about his nervousness because everything here was so new for him. I could sense how important it was for him to have at least the consistency of art therapy to release his feelings.

For the following session I met him on the day-treatment unit, where he was getting his iv-immunosuppressive medication. I sensed his nervousness and insecurity. He was very irritable and did not know what do draw. I suggested doing a drawing about his actual feelings. He asked for more concrete help, and within my own embarrassment I suggested another bridge drawing. He liked this idea and started right away with a pencil drawing (Figure 3.15: Bridge Drawing, pencil drawing by Abdul, 16 years).

At the end of the session, I asked him for some associations. He told me that the bridge's direction was from the left to the right side and was going over a huge river. It was a full-moon night and there were four streetlights on the bridge (perhaps symbolizing his supportive family?). He was already on the bridge, but still at the very end of it and in the shadow of a huge protective tree. When I asked him about the second person in the boat, he said: "He is crazy. He's risking his life by using this small boat in the middle of the night, in this dark water of this huge river." I wondered if it represented another part of himself adventuring into the depth of his unconsciousness.

The bridge was strong, similar to the very first one (Plate 2, p. 45), but this time had railings for safety reasons. Abdul obviously had managed to go onto the bridge, but was still at the very beginning. The bridge was heading to nowhere. Obviously, he realized that transplantation was not the final solution, that there was still a long way to go, and that his future was still very unclear.

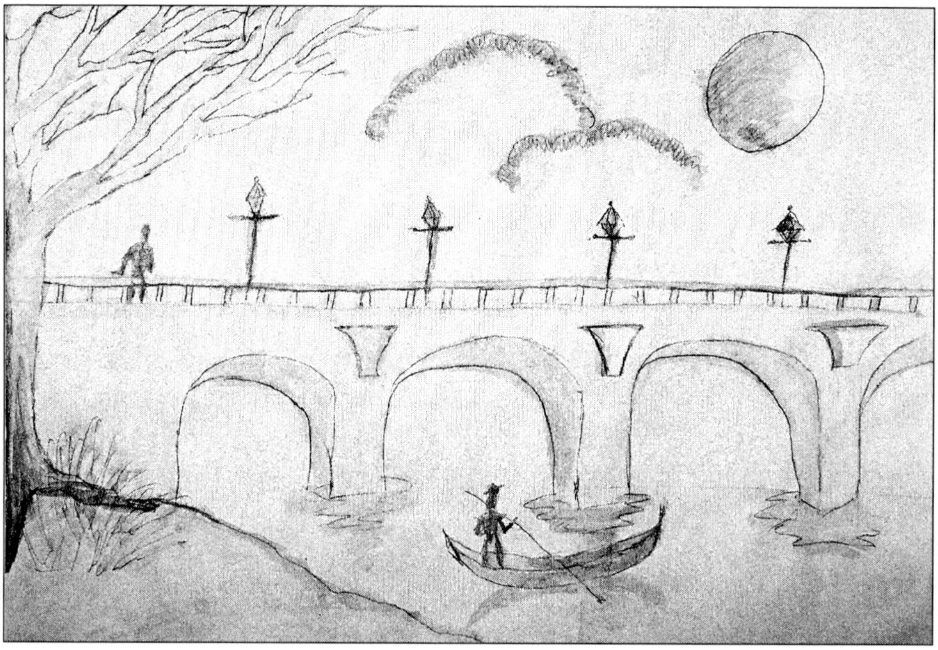

Figure 3.15. Bridge Drawing, pencil drawing by Abdul, 16 years.

At the following session he was less nervous, but still confused. I could sense that he needed to talk and to report on his medical condition and treatments. Everything was fine. He obviously needed to share with somebody the huge responsibility he had to bear. While he was talking he did a pencil drawing (Figure 3.16: "da Vinci's Anatomical Wheel," pencil drawing by Abdul, 16 years).

He first drew an upright, standing, faceless human figure with hanging arms and extraordinarily small hands. Then he added an elevated set of arms, and then another set. The same happened with the legs. When he was done I asked for his associations, and he told me about da Vinci's wheel of anatomical proportions. He added that he greatly admired it.

But because Abdul's drawing did not contain the circle that gave shape to Da Vinci's famous drawing, my own associations with his drawing led me to wonder if his figure was more about a string puppet without the guidance and support of strings, or perhaps a parachute jumper who's parachute had not opened yet, or maybe even the uncoordinated movements of a person who was learning to swim. Somehow, I sensed helplessness in his struggle to become adjusted to an unknown environment. Was he expressing his conflict about his body, about the mutilation of his body?

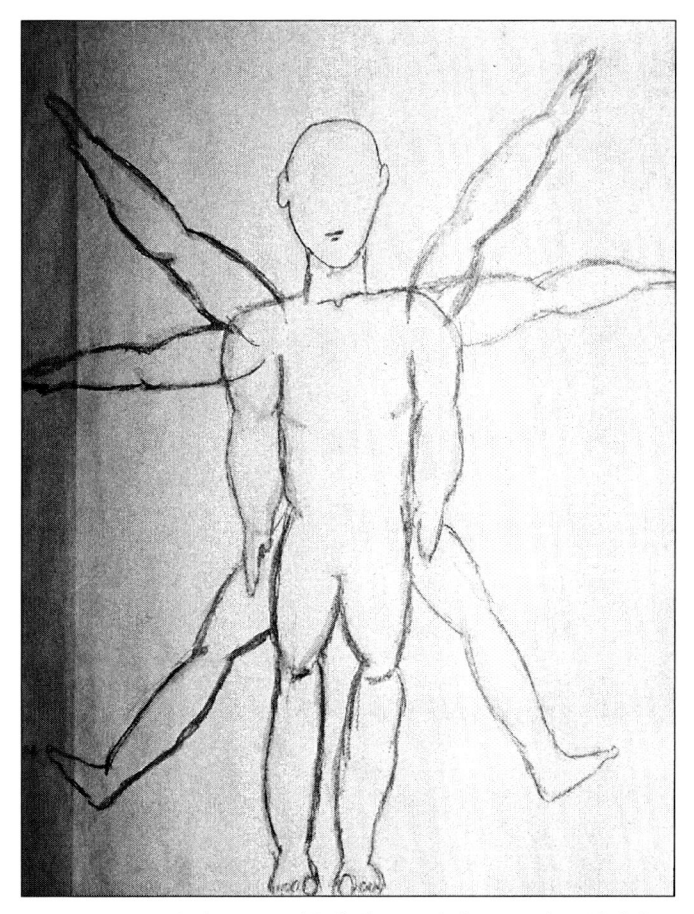

Figure 3.16. *Da Vinci's Anatomical Wheel*, pencil drawing by Abdul, 16 years.

Over the course of the following weeks he seemed to regain some of his self-confidence. He appeared to be less tense and more contained. For one of these sessions he was waiting for me in the Nephrology outpatient area. It was the session at which we had to start termination. Due to his excellent physical condition, he only had to come for follow-up appointments every other week. The next step would be to stretch the appointments to once a month, which would most likely mean the end of the art therapy program for Abdul.

Choosing water-soluble pencil, he did not know right away what to draw. But then he declared: "I know you would like me to draw a landscape. Today you should get it!" (Figure 3.17: "My Landscape," pencil drawing by Abdul, 16 years).

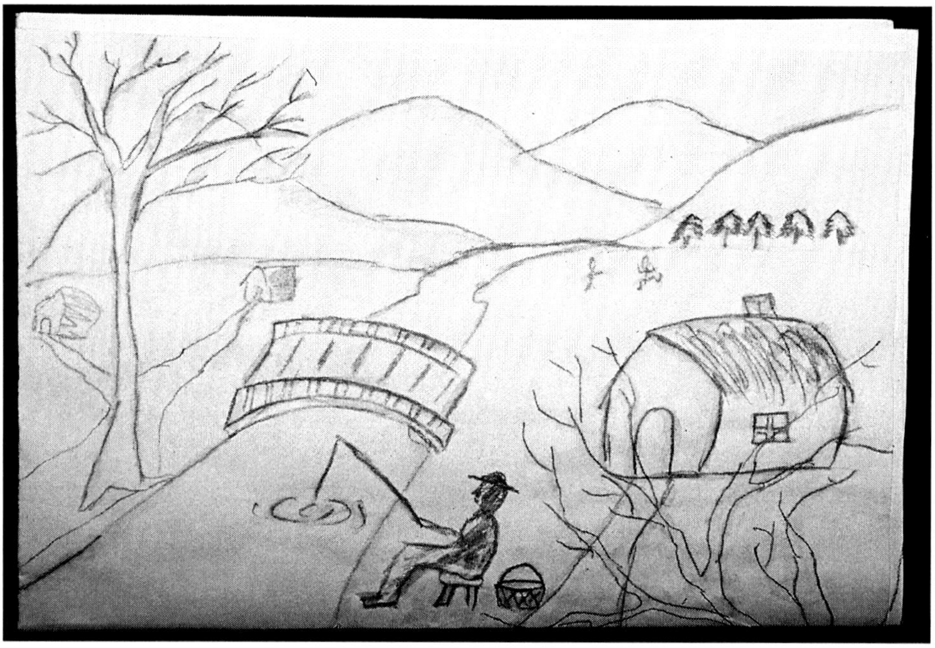

Figure 3.17. *My Landscape*, pencil drawing by Abdul, 16 years.

He folded the big paper twice and started to draw a landscape with remarkable similarities to the second picture he had done at the very beginning of art therapy (Plate 1, p. 45). This time, though, there was also a bridge and a human figure with his house. The river seemed to be tamed now and not flooding anymore. When I asked him where he would be in this picture, he added a hat onto the fisherman's head and answered: "Here, although I don't like fish at all."

While he was drawing, he asked me what I worked at back home and why I wouldn't do the same job here. "It's not so easy," was my short answer. His question was obviously a starting point for sharing. Now he released his frustration, about how this country recruited people from abroad, and then didn't offer them appropriate and decent jobs just because they were foreigners, and how much his family life suffers because of the working shifts, and how often he would feel alone. I asked him about friends. He told me that he had one Spanish, two Jamaican and only one Caucasian friend, really good friends! He added that he did not have a lot of contact with his school peers because they were all into drugs and smoking, and he did not want to deal with that. "I would like to have reliable friends who like to study and to learn things to become smart."

Although he obviously was able now to connect the two cultures (symbolized by the two connected river shores), his picture definitively mirrors his loneliness and isolation.

When we met for the following session he did not know what to do. So I suggested that he have a look at his landscape again. I opened the double-folded paper once, and he then decided to add more to the picture (Figure 3.18: "My Landscape," continuation of pencil drawing by Abdul, 16 years).

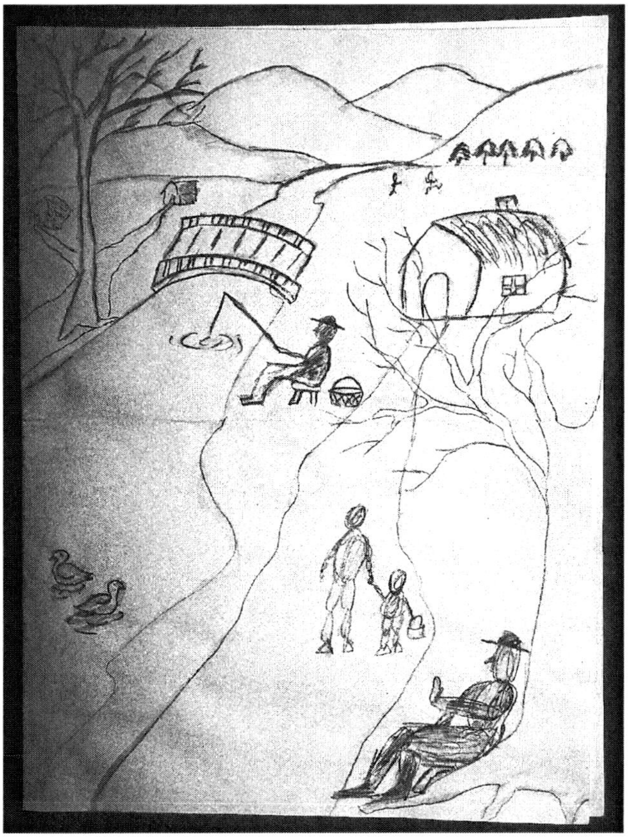

Figure 3.18. *My Landscape*, continuation of pencil drawing by Abdul, 16 years.

He extended the river. Under a huge tree there was a human figure with the same features as the fisherman. He told me that it was an old man waving to his old friend who was walking with his grandson. The season was early spring, the trees would sprout soon. He did not give me more associations.

I wondered about the old man's sign. To me, it was more about keeping other people distant. Was this a metaphor for Abdul's ambivalence during all these weeks: needing to be intimate, but separate and independent at the same time? And what about grandfather and grandson? Were these the two parts of himself, representing his past and future, while the sitting man was more the present? Was that another symbol for the search for his identity? Or was it more a metaphor for the child within himself, still dependent on a nurturing caregiver and in need for a secure attachment?

He started the next session by spontaneously opening the paper of his landscape again. Immediately he started to extend it further (Figure 3.19: "My Landscape," continuation of pencil drawing by Abdul, 16 years).

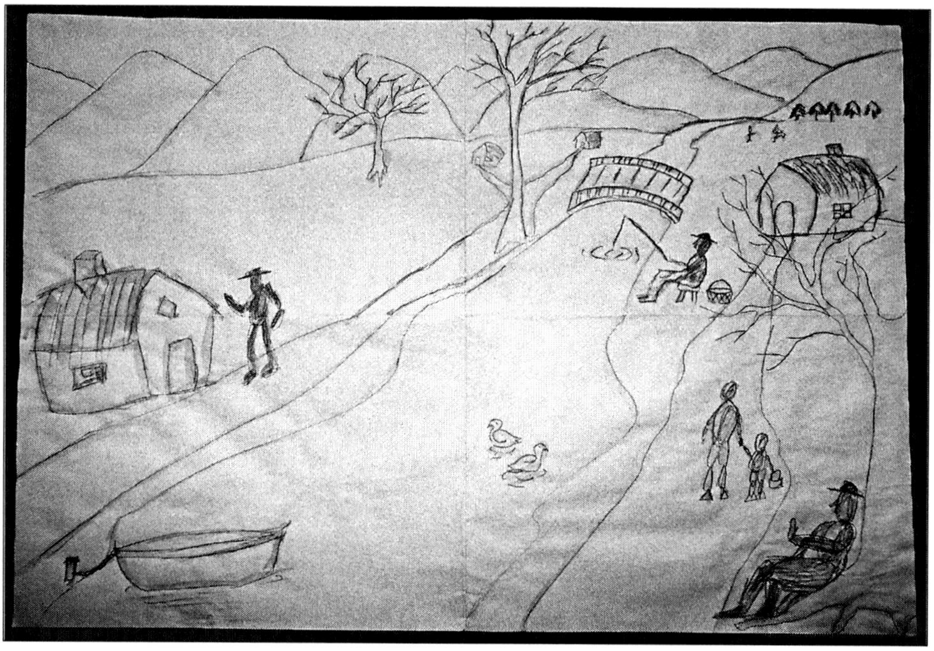

Figure 3.19. *My Landscape*, continuation of pencil drawing by Abdul, 16 years.

Again the man with the typical features reappeared walking on the left (past related) side of the river. There was a boat tied up after it had crossed the river back again. And again this striking loneliness!

He had no time to give me associations. While he was drawing, he told me about his first day back at school with his class, and how nice was their welcome for him. They all told him how much he had changed. He was now, they said, a mature adult man. To Abdul, though, his classmates all looked the same. Then he started to tell me about his long-term plans. He would graduate after grade 12 next year, and then he would start studying social sciences. Later, he would add environmental science and political science at university, and then enter law school. He was obviously exploring his future possibilities, and his academic ambitions were reactivated. I wondered why he was finishing his drawing at the left river side (related to the past), while he told me about his future.

The gradual development of his landscape seemed to be his way to wrap-up what had happened over the last few months – Abdul's way of termination.

At the beginning of the second last session I started off by reminding him that we were approaching the end of the art therapy program. He apparently did not care, or at least he did not show any reactions. I was wondering if he was denying his feelings about termination.

On the table we worked at, he found a drawing another child had done of a totem pole. What did it represent, he asked? Surprisingly, he didn't know anything about totem poles, so I gave him some explanations. He liked the idea and decided to draw his own totem pole to put in front of his own room (Figure 3.20: "My Totem Pole," pencil drawing by Abdul, 16 years). This time, he gave me his associations right away. The top figure was a horned, ugly face to scare bad ghosts, followed by two pet-mascots for good luck, followed by a horizontal decoration to make the whole thing more human-like, followed by an ancient Egyptian cross (symbol for eternal life) that he learned about at school (perhaps a metaphor for his education, which he very much enjoyed?), followed by a vulture-ninja for protection, followed by the Indian national logo, "the four lions," heading in the four directions (symbol for his Indian background) and finally grounded by three richly decorated legs in Indian style (symbol for his own Indian roots). How better could he summarize all his qualities and needs?

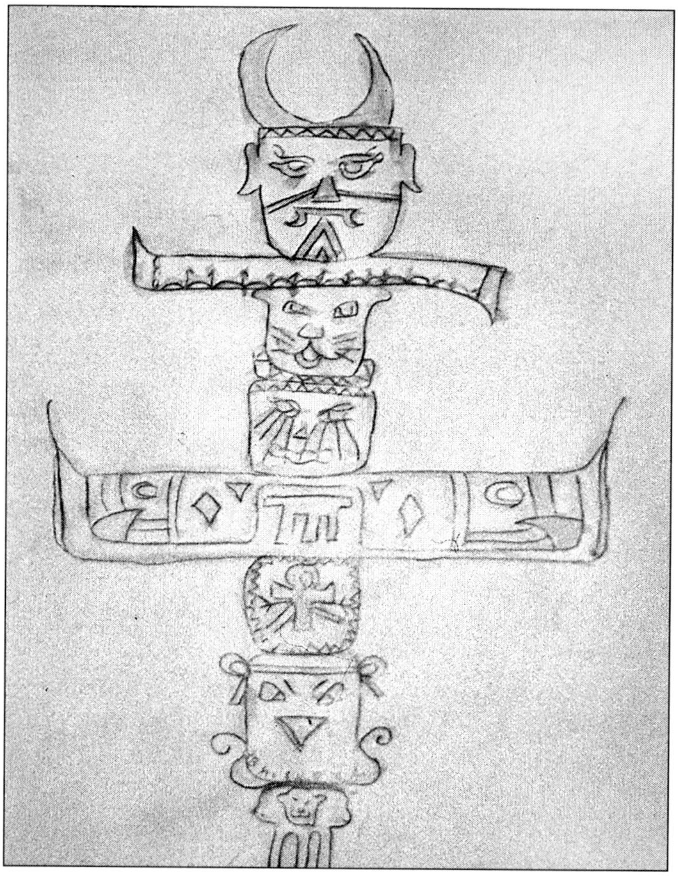

Figure 3.20. *My Totem Pole*, pencil drawing by Abdul, 16 years.

That day it was hard to finish the session and I gave him extra time because we met only every second week. He first told me about his new hobby: gardening. His parents had given him the responsibility for the garden. He enjoyed his new job and was growing a lot of Indian spices and herbs and vegetables.

Before he left, he told me about his favorite class: parenting! Together we laughed, reminding each other how upset he was at the beginning of this class some months ago, when he was still on hemodialysis. He told me about all the psychological developmental stages a child had to go through, adding practical examples of his own life, acknowledging his parents' qualities and struggles. He finished this lecture with an Indian saying: "The mother who cares for her child too much, will make it sick." I wondered if he was relating that to his life as well.

Finally, he left the session by uttering the English saying: "It is better to light a candle than to curse the darkness." I wondered about all these sayings that day: Was that the way he kept himself contained by giving himself structure during termination?

During the last session we reviewed his folder with all the artwork he produced over the last nine months. The goal was to decide, which Abdul wanted to take home, and with which he was not comfortable enough to take it home. Making comments about each single piece Abdul seemed to connect all sorts of memories. It was like a journey through a visual diary. There were not pieces he did not feel comfortable with. Apparently all were equally important for this journey of development. Finally he closed the folder and handed it to me with the words: "That's for you. You should have all my work. Not because I could not take it home. But because you deserve it. What I needed to learn from my artwork, I am carrying deep within myself. I don't need the paper anymore. But you should have it as a thank you for what you have done for me. Maybe my folder can help other kids to master their difficulties." Of course I was totally overwhelmed and did not know what to answer right away. In my embarrassment I double-checked with him, if he would not regret this step later. But he was convinced to do the right thing. In my thinking as a therapist I was wondering about other reasons for not wanting to take home his artwork, but could not come up with any conclusions, even in discussing with my supervisor. Was he just trying reminding me of him, as he would not forget me? Or did he want to be as important to me, as I was for him?

SUMMARY

Sixteen-year-old Abdul was very well able to connect with me. Over the period of the nine months of treatment, his behavior towards me changed from polite defensive, over to defiant rejection with passive aggression, and into a friendly collegial interaction. After the initial phase of forming a trustful working alliance he was able to let fall the censorship of aesthetics, and to use his art to explore his feelings, issues and conflicts related to his developmental stage and to his physical illness, and finally, to integrate his new acquaintances into his identity.

5. Jayson, Male, 13 Years

Description of the Client

Jayson is a short and chubby 13-year-old teenager of Indian origin. He looks younger than his age, and his face has a childlike, helpless expression. He has striking big black eyes in deep eye sockets, which give him an unhealthy appearance. When he's in an upright position one becomes aware of his very short and crooked legs. When he walks, his gait shows a labored and inhomogeneous pattern. As a result, he has difficulties keeping his balance. These gross motor disturbances were caused by his severe osteoporosis.

Jayson is an adolescent of average intelligence. He is in grade seven and has age-appropriate academic skills even though he has had frequent absences right from the time he started school because of his chronic physical illness. He has a moderate curiosity and often lacked motivation and, therefore, liked to spend a lot of time in front of the TV or the computer playing the same games over and over again in order to distract himself. Since he wasn't able to participate in team sports, he seemed to choose passive over active entertainment.

He was not a talker at all, and he would never disclose any thoughts or feelings. His behavior was withdrawn and reserved. He rarely would share anything, not even happy events. It was as if he couldn't trust anybody. His mood was even, with a good portion of underlying sadness, which he tried to hide with a weak smile on his face, reminiscent of a mask. He had good impulse control and would never show his anger or frustration openly. He was more of a passive-aggressive type of personality, showing avoidance when angry or annoyed.

He had poor communication skills, and often displayed an absent face, although I was sure he was listening attentively. He seemed to know his limitations and never risked going beyond them in order to avoid the need for help or any kind of dependence. In doing art together, we rarely reached the point at which we had a comfortable back and forth relationship, neither on a verbal or non-verbal basis. Since he was not regularly able to attend school and because he spent a lot of time at the hospital and did not have terribly good social skills, he didn't have many opportunities in which to develop social contacts. Beside his good relationships with his cousins, he seemed to be quite isolated.

He showed a very narrow range of interests. Sports seemed to be his favorite. He very rarely followed directives. He made me list several suggestions and than chose something I did not mention in order to keep control and a sense of autonomy.

Jayson's strongest defense mechanism was withdrawal into passive-aggression, especially when he had to deal with anger and aggression. These negative feelings seemed to be intolerable to him and needed to be either displaced or kept under control in another way. Another strong defense mechanism was his escape into physical symptoms related to his illness. Often it was very difficult to know if he had organic reasons for a headache or dizziness (high/low blood pressure, etc.), or if it was kind of a somatization of inner conflicts in order to escape doing art, fearing the loss of control over his emotions. (Here I want to make a strict differentiation to "simulation," which to me has a conscious component.)

Art therapy with Jayson was different than it was with other clients. With them, therapist and client managed to form a mutual attachment. But Jayson and I never did build a trustful working alliance. In fact, I started to wonder about his ability to form attachments with anybody, even his own mother. The whole program with Jayson was characterized by week-long interruptions due to resistance and avoidance, although I tried to be as consistent and as flexible as possible in looking after him and arranging appointments. I tried to give him as much control as possible, not only in terms of art material, techniques and themes, but also in scheduling. Sometimes I had the feeling he was taking advantage of me and was trying to provoke me, though I also realized that some of these actions were prompted by his poor physical condition.

Even though Jayson volunteered for the program, he was not terribly engaged by it, and he never asked for help. He always performed with a frozen smile on his lips, never showing emotions, neither good nor bad. I often felt like a spectator in front of a stage, where a drama was happening behind closed curtains, making it impossible for me to participate.

Often I had another association: I felt like I had been left out in the rain, while standing in front of a closed door of a house in which lights proved that there was life inside. Thinking back to these moments, I now know that it was perhaps about "projective identification," and that I was picking up on his feelings of abandonment, of being excluded from life.

Social History

Both parents were of Indian origin. The mother was born and grew up in North America with her family and her two brothers. The father had immigrated at the age of 17 years. They had met here, although their families already had a connection back in India, and had arranged the marriage when Jayson's parents were still children. When Jayson was 10 years old, his father died unexpectedly of a stroke. He left behind his young wife with two children – Jayson and his 8-year-old sister. Neither the mother, nor the children, nor the whole family together were able to go through appropriate grief work. Their father still lived like a ghost among them. It was a situation that added to Jayson's problems in coping with life.

Fortunately, the mother had her extended family, which included her mother and two brothers, living in the vicinity, which helped her a lot in supporting and caring for her two kids. She had a part-time job as a hairdresser. When she and Jayson finally started with nightly home dialysis, Jayson's family was allowed to move into the house of one of the maternal uncles, and to install the machine there.

Jayson was a wanted child. Pregnancy and delivery, as well as the first years of development were uneventful, with normal developmental milestones. After the age of five years, when his kidney problems started, Jayson suffered more and more developmental delays in different areas. His physical growth curve slowed down, he started his academic career with frequent absences from school right from the beginning, and he had difficulties in developing appropriate social skills and building a supportive circle of good friends. Unlike his classmates, he was never able to go to school on a regular basis. Fortunately, he was well-embedded in his extended family on his mother's side, and had good relationships with his uncles and cousins. After his father's death these relationships became even more important for him. He did not seem to be really attached to his sister.

I tried over and over again to approach his mother and to arrange an appointment. However, she somehow showed the same avoidant behavior as her son did. She never showed up for interviews. I got all the information about Jayson's life from his social worker. Questions about how Jayson was as a young child before his adolescence, what kind of family dynamics were active, how Jayson's relationship with his father was, and how actively he would invest in peer relationships and friendships, will remain unanswered.

Medical History

From birth Jayson developed normally and had strong health. His kidney problems started at the age of five, when he developed "Focal Glomerulosclerosis," a disease resulting in the destruction of the kidneys by circulating auto-antibodies. Gradually, both kidneys gave up their function. Due to a severe accompanying Nephrotic Syndrome (and therefore an uncontrollable loss of protein through the filtration defect of the kidneys), he had to have both his kidneys removed. Therefore, he became permanently dependent on regular kidney replacement therapy by around the age of six.

His physicians first tried to treat him with peritoneal dialysis. Due to a fungal peritonitis with pancreatitis (a very severe and potentially life-threatening condition) caused by unsterile handling of the electrolyte solution, peritoneal dialysis had to be changed to hemodialysis. After his father's death, Jayson suffered from a severe, life-threatening bacterial sepsis, requiring the removal and replacement of his hemodialysis catheter.

During the following four years, he had two kidney transplantations and two rejections due to non-compliance in taking the immunosuppressive medication. As a result, he was back on hemodialysis.

Due to poor compliance in medication, he also had a severe osteoporosis (insufficient intake of calcium) with marked valgus deformity of his legs. Furthermore, his non-compliance in medication and restriction of salt and fluid intake had resulted in uncontrollable hypertension, with consecutive headaches and dizziness (e.g., after his mother had hidden the salt, he ate "Ajax" behind his mother's back, knowing that this detergent contains salt!). Each week he needed additional hemodialysis treatment sessions because of his non-compliance. As a result, he was usually on hemodialysis 4–5 times a week, for four hours per treatment.

Over the years – nobody knew when exactly – Jayson started to gradually develop a so-called Pica-disease, in which he would eat all kinds of foam rubber by opening pillows, mattresses and cushions of sofas and picking out the material. Pica is an eating disorder defined as the persistent eating of non-nutritive substances for a period of at least one month at an age in which this behavior is developmentally inappropriate. Although the etiology of this disturbance is unknown, several hypotheses try to explain this phenomenon. They range from psychosocial causes to causes of purely biochemical origin. The list of hypothetical causes includes: (1) nutritional deficiencies (e.g., deficiency or absence of iron, calcium, zinc, etc.); (2) underlying biochemical disorders (e.g., association with iron deficiency and other pathophysiologic states with decreased activity of certain neurotransmitters (dopamine) in the brain, which in turns maintains pica behavior); (3) cultural and familial factors (e.g., parental role modeling, etc.); (4) psychosocial stress (e.g., maternal deprivation, parental separation, parental neglect, child abuse, etc.); (5) low socioeconomic status (e.g., malnutrition and hunger, lack of parental supervision, etc.); and finally, (6) non-discriminating oral behavior (e.g., inability to discriminate between food and non-food items in mental retardation) (Ellis, 2002).

In Jayson's case numerous blood tests and examinations had been completed, but none offered any organic explanation for his behavior. Therefore, a psychosocial issue seemed to be the most likely cause.

Towards the end of the art therapy program, Jayson and his mother started training on how to manage and run a dialysis machine at home, six nights a week while he was sleeping. The training for this new circumstance turned out to be a difficult time for the two of them, especially for Jayson. He obviously had a hard time taking on this huge responsibility, and trying to prove his reliability and compliance. He apparently also had a hard time in fully trusting his mother since over the years she, at times, had been just as non-compliant as he had been regarding treatment.

The numerous scars that covered Jayson's body reminded one not only of his long history of suffering, but also of the additional impact they must have had on his self-esteem. I was asked to work with Jayson by his social worker. The hope was that art therapy could help him to gain more self-confidence, to strengthen his self-esteem, and to help him to become aware of the importance of a good compliance. Our art therapy program of 27 sessions over nine months was characterized by a lot of resistance and avoidance, but never total rejection.

Art Therapy Process and Artwork

The art therapy program with Jayson, which lasted for 27 sessions over a period of nine months, was characterized by short episodes of close work, interrupted by rejection and avoidance due to resistance.

I was introduced to Jayson and his very young-looking mother by the social worker a week before I started to work with him. When I met Jayson for the first time, I found him looking very tired and lying flat supine. When I asked him if he felt like doing something, he answered in a low voice: "Yes, but my machine doesn't tolerate my sitting position." That was how I learned about his troubles with his central line. During the whole art therapy program of nine months, he had problems with the line, which often required that he lie flat on his back. Not being allowed to sit during hemodialysis was another huge restriction for Jayson, and a big disadvantage for the process of art therapy. In these cases, I tried to give him another chance to have his session the same week whenever it was possible. However, three days after our first meeting, his line was still not working properly. So we spent a lot of time just talking in regard to what art therapy was all about, confidentiality, the offer of art material, and so forth.

The following week when I met him he was in a sitting position. He was waiting for me, ready to do art. He chose pencil and pencil crayons and right away started to decorate the cover of his folder by carefully drawing an outline first, and then coloring it with crayons. (Figure 3.21: "My Flags," pencil crayon by Jayson, 13 years).

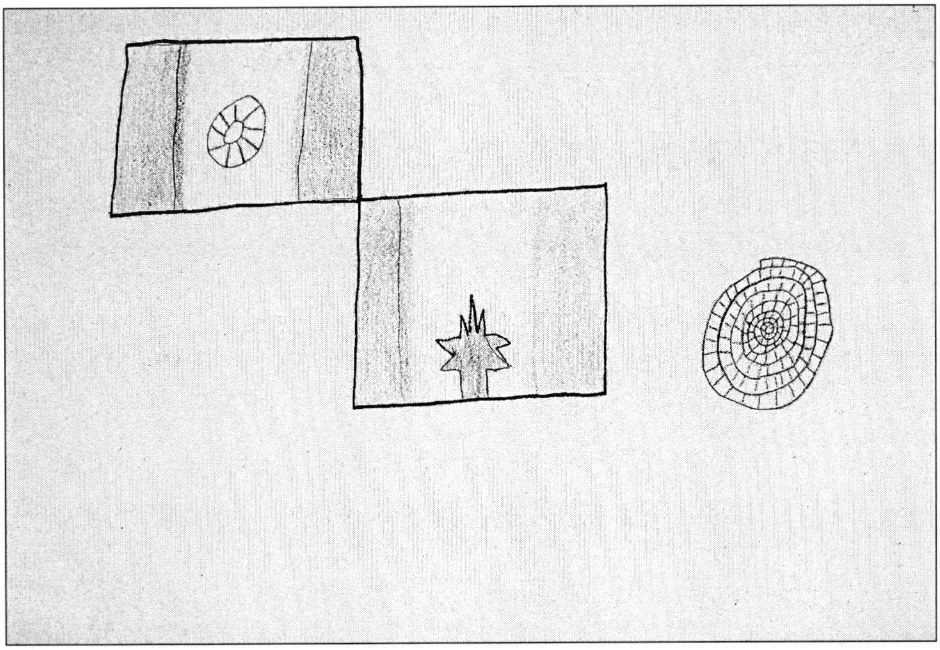

Figure 3.21. *My Flags*, pencil crayon drawing by Jayson, 13 years.

While he was drawing he talked only sporadically, commenting on the two flags: the Indian to the left, the Canadian on the right. He pointed out that both his parents were Indian, but that he was Canadian. Then he quickly added a spiral in black crayon, developing the line from the center to the outside, but adding spikes from the outside inwards. He did not want to give me any associations for it. However, to me it looked like a spider web or a maze, something to be trapped in.

For several sessions we were not able to work together because of the poor function of his central line He had to lie flat and was not allowed to use his right arm, which meant even more restrictions. During one session when he was totally immobilized, the Bingo program was on the *Sick Kids* TV Channel. Jayson was very disappointed at not being able to participate. So I suggested that I help him and together we won a big book about games. He was totally excited. Even if it was not about doing art, I was hoping to establish a trustful working alliance.

At the following session his line was working properly, which allowed Jayson to make art. He seemed to be keen on showing me all the artistic special effects he had learned at school. First he asked for paint (Figure 3.22: "The Rainbow," watercolor by Jayson, 13 years). He painted vertical lines in different colors, and then while it was still wet, folded the paper in half. With a mysterious smile he unfolded the paper again and showed me the result. He seemed to be proud of his good idea, although he was annoyed by all the white gaps in between the color stripes. He did not give me any associations, but titled it "The Rainbow." I had two responses: that it gave off a strong nice and colorful feeling; and that it was like a set of closed curtains, behind which anything could be hidden. Was he bothered by the gaps because they could allow seeing behind the scenes?

Fully in action, he switched to oil pastels and black paint. Without talking, he spontaneously covered the paper with vertical stripes in different colors in oil pastels, then covered it with black paint. Finally, he started to scratch into the black paint and to write his full name. While he was working, his machine sounded an alarm because the blood flow was not high enough, so he had to interrupt his artwork and take a semi-sitting position. He was very disappointed and made a face. So I suggested we look for a solution that would allow him to continue his work. I organized a big book as a surface to work on his knees to replace the table while being prone. While he was painting I was holding the cup of water and the black paint in reachable distance. If he appreciated this help, he was not able to show it. However, he seemed to enjoy being able to finish his piece. For a while we talked about the troubles with his line and he was able to share and release some of his frustrations about it.

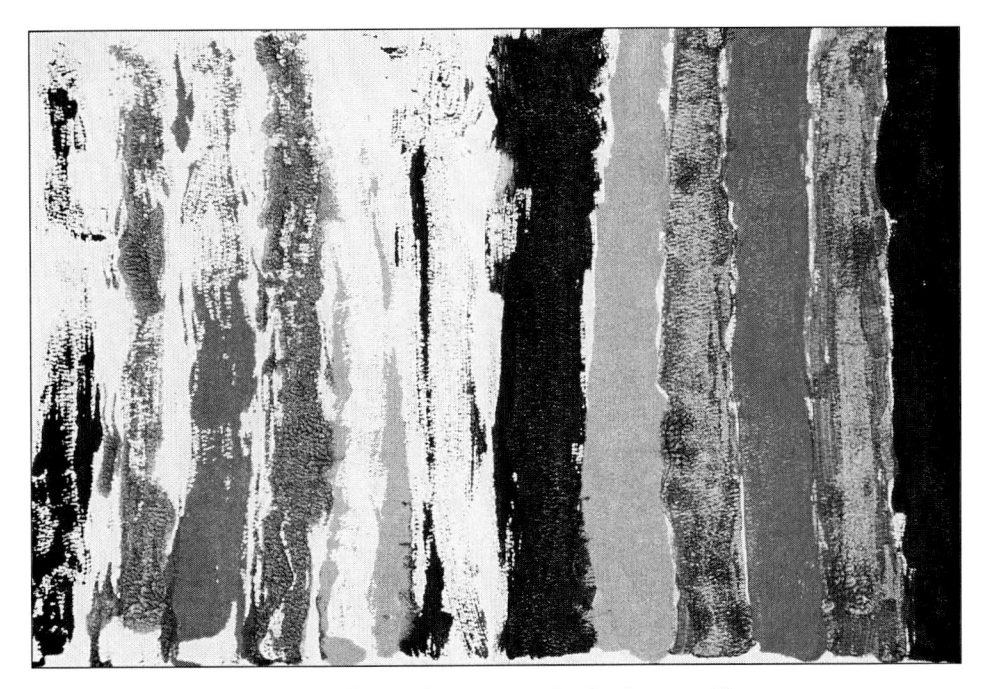

Figure 3.22. *The Rainbow*, watercolor by Jayson, 13 years.

While sitting close to him during his painting I became overwhelmed by my own inner sadness and I wondered if I had picked up on his inner sadness (projective identification). Having a final look at his black picture with his small scratched name lost in darkness I had the feeling of even more layers of heavier curtains hiding something unbearable, allowing only the pure fact of his name to appear. The second feeling I had was the sensation of falling short – I felt like I was sitting in front of a stage knowing that behind the closed curtains a probably very dramatic play was taking place.

For the whole of the following week there was no way we could do some art. When I looked for him at the beginning of the week, I found him as an inpatient. He had to be hospitalized by ambulance because of a "hypertensive crisis," a state in which the blood pressure becomes almost uncontrollably high; in these cases, the risk of a cerebral hemorrhage is extremely high. He had caused this critical stage by drinking over 5 liters of fluid over the weekend.

For the rest of the week I visited him several times, just to sit and chat or to play some sort of game for about 15–20 minutes. During this week he was very reserved and depressed, and did not want to talk about anything related to his disease. Obviously, he was fearing more reproaches. I had the impression that he just needed some distraction for a little while.

Finally, the week after, he was fine again, and his line was working perfectly. Nevertheless he seemed unmotivated, and his non-verbal signals were this: He would tolerate me today, but he wouldn't share anything at all. Avoiding any eye contact, he seemed reluctant to interact with me in any kind of way.

He chose paint and started to mix some brown (Figure 3.23: "Fast Flying Balls," watercolor by Jayson, 13 years). Then, without making pencil outlines first, he started to paint all kinds of balls: a football, a baseball, a soccer ball, a basketball, a golf ball and a hockey puck. All the balls were in high motion, heading to the right side (related to the future), all with fire-like rockets to underline the high speed. I asked him for his associations, and he told me that all the balls were flying like rockets because somebody kicked them really hard. He did not want to tell me more.

In this picture I could feel his frustration and anger to a full extent. These balls had the aspect of missiles and a violent content. Was he shooting at his future, trying to kill it? At the same time, all these balls represented the games he was dreaming of but was not allowed to play due to being connected to his central line.

At the beginning of the following week his line did not work again. He was angry, depressed and frustrated. I visited him each day when he was on hemodialysis for two reasons – one was to offer him an opportunity to release his frustration through talking or being distracted through games; the other was to make sure we would not miss a day in which he could do some art.

When I found him at the end of the week, his line was finally working again. Although he knew I would come at a certain time, he had started a computer game. When I met him, he seemed to be annoyed by my presence. Although he could sit he did not want to be interrupted in his computer game just for doing art. He explained to me that he was not an artist at all, and didn't really like to draw and paint. I told him again about art therapy, and that one did not have to be an artist in order to do it. I also told him that since his participation was on a voluntary basis, he had the option of dropping out at any point. Suddenly I could feel that his attitude was not directly related to art therapy at all. Up until now he had never uttered a single word about wanting to stop. I got the feeling that his behaviour was more about having a sense of control over the situation, about having the right to make his own decisions, even if it was only about art therapy.

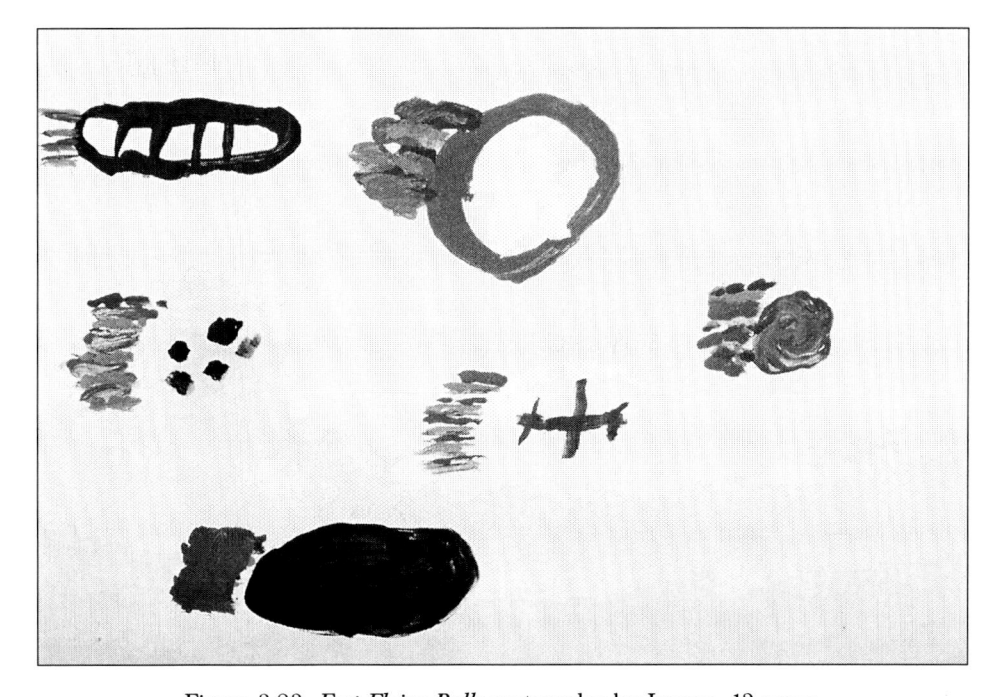

Figure 3.23. *Fast Flying Balls*, watercolor by Jayson, 13 years.

At the following session his line was working properly. I found him sitting on his small table and sticking stickers onto his school folder. That made me suggest that he make a collage. He seemed to be interested in this suggestion and he started looking through the image collection right away. He then decided to make two collages with his favorite themes: one of sports and one of animals, starting with the sports (Plate 5 "Sports," collage by Jayson, 13 years, p. 47). While he was arranging and gluing, we talked about his favorite sport, which was baseball, and how he played it with friends in his spare time. I wondered if he was telling me about a wish or a dream, knowing that he had almost no spare time, and few social contacts outside of his family. On top of everything, he was not allowed to play team games due to his very fragile central line.

Then he decided to start the animal collage. Although we were running out of time, I decided to give him additional time and the control over ending the session. At the very beginning, he asked me for help in taping two white papers together, knowing that this collage would become very big. Then he started again to select, cut and arrange animals (Figure 3.24: "Animals," collage by Jayson, 13 years).

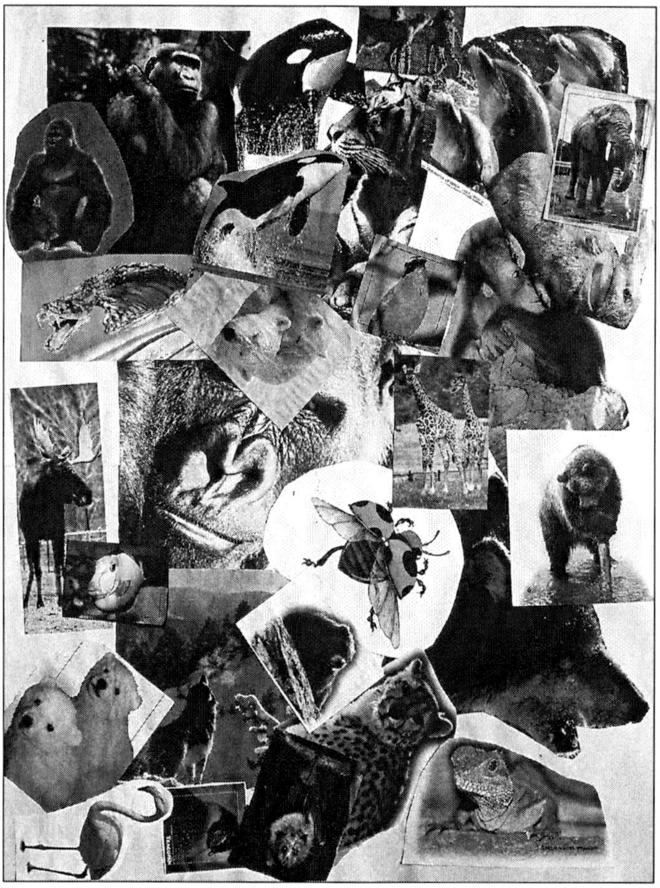

Figure 3.24. *Animals*, collage by Jayson, 13 years.

I was surprised by how uncontrolled and unplanned the collage became. Jayson overlapped images, turned them upside down, and covered dominant parts of images (e.g. eyes of a face) with another image, but always leaving some free space here and there. While he was working, we talked about his favorite animals: mainly dogs, but also dolphins and whales (all animals which live in clearly structured groups, and perhaps representing his wish for reliable friendship) – and bugs as well! I discovered some powerful animals like tigers, bears and wolves (representing his wish for protection?). It was a loose, but superficial conversation. For the first time I had the feeling that we were able to connect to each other on a deeper level by developing a nice teamwork. As a whole image, the animal collage seemed to be well balanced, although somehow chaotic and without clear orientation. The most striking thing was a big flying ladybug located almost in the center of the page. Leaving a lot of white paper around the bug, Jayson gave it the sense to fly through a suggested hole in the paper. Showing its back, it was as if the bug would leave the turmoil around him by moving to the background, or leaving the scene through a back door. Was that Jayson's unconscious wish – to leave the scene of all the turmoil and chaos around him? At the same time this nice ladybug showed such a fragility, Jayson's own vulnerability?

However, I was very surprised about the change in Jayson after the last session, at which he seemed to reject me totally. We seemed to have discovered the appropriate means for him.

He started the following session by checking his previous collages, showing big pleasure or pride in his creations. Then he immediately wanted to add more images to his first sports collage. He flipped through the image collection and selected all the sports and car images he could find. He then asked me to put the car images into his folder in order to save them for next time, since today he was planning to finish his first sport collage. First, he cut all the images, making clear decisions about which way to cut them (rectangular or outline). Then he put all the images down without gluing them, trying different options, changing interactions and positions until he was fully satisfied. Then he decided that now it was "gluing time." He was greatly enjoying this process and worked with intense concentration, seldom talking (Figure 3.25: "Sports," detail of the collage by Jayson, 13 years).

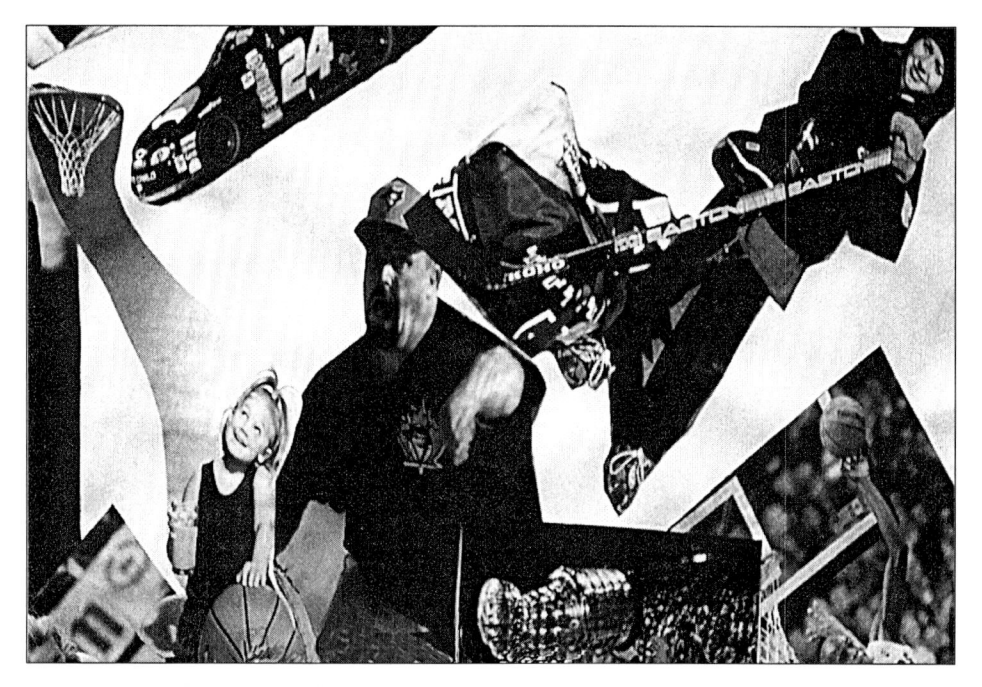

Figure 3.25. *Sports*, detail of the collage by Jayson, 13 years.

The first striking thing was his choice of a small boy holding a long hockey stick overlapping the head of a strong American football player, and apparently trying to hit the head of this big, powerful guy. Was this scene representing his anger and frustration while at the same time showing his vulnerability?

The second striking thing was his choice of a little girl kneeling behind a huge basketball, holding a big glass of orange juice in her right hand and aiming with her eyes at a distant basket in the blue sky. Jayson glued her in the center of the page, which gave a special meaning to this scene. The girl is laughing and seems to be confident that she will succeed at hitting the distant basket with the right energy. With her orange juice, the metaphor for fluid, which is a permanent issue in Jayson's non-compliance in diet, was this little girl a symbol for opposition, for defiance? On the one hand, her longing gaze could symbolize his wish to be strong enough to contain himself, in order to be able to respect the restriction of a certain amount of fluid intake per day? On the other hand, she has a fragile appearance, symbolizing his own vulnerability. Was this scene just trying to show us that he was simply too weak for this overwhelming task of showing compliance and taking over responsibility?

Again we had an interesting teamwork, although this time without a lot of verbal sharing. By the end of the session his line started to make troubles again, but he wanted to finish his collage despite his laying-flat position. He told me exactly how to cut the images (e.g., by respecting the rectangular shape of the photograph, or by cutting the outlines of the figure in question). After I put some glue onto the back of the image, he put it down, choosing the appropriate placement. This teamwork obviously allowed him to move between himself and the outside, creating a supportive and responsive flow between me (representing the outside support) and his emotional world. This collage became the link.

For the following session he was waiting for me and wanted to start right away with a new collage (Plate 6: "Sports II," p. 47, and Figure 3.26: detail of the collage "Sports II" by Jayson, 13 years). This time he asked for a really huge piece of paper. He was very keen on looking through the image collection. Then he started to cut, arrange and glue down images. This time he seemed to carefully plan the placements of the images by holding them onto different spots, and then observing the image through squeezed eyes. For the whole session, he was working with great, silent concentration. He seemed to put the pictures in a clearly defined correlation to one another.

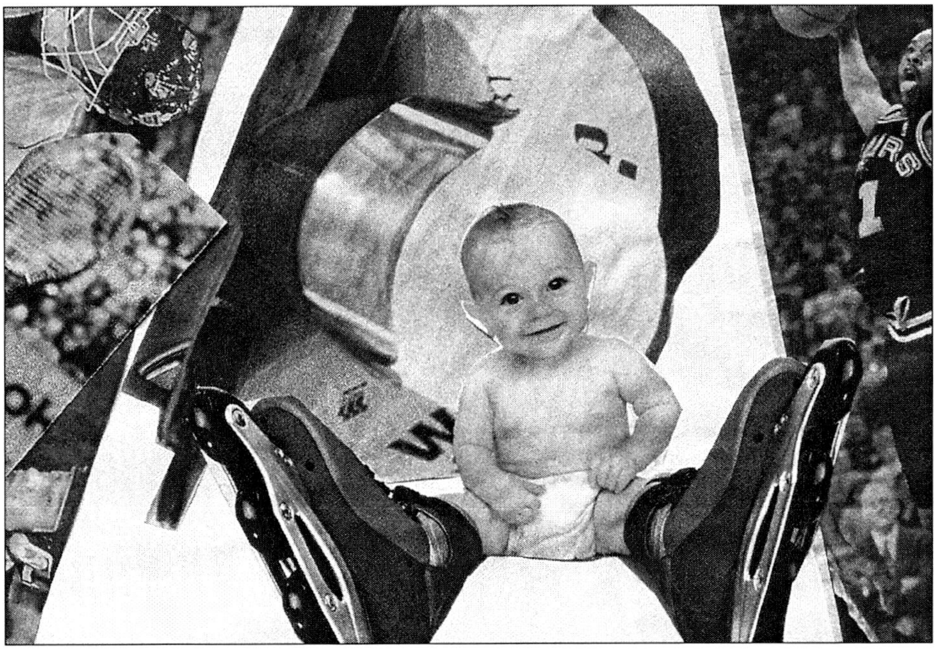

Figure 3.26. *Sports II*, detail of the collage by Jayson, 13 years.

The striking thing was his choice of a sitting toddler in diapers, wearing oversized roller blades. He positioned this image in the low center, giving it a special meaning. Whereas all around this toddler there were a lot of strong men fighting in team sports, his appearance is one of an alien. To me this image could be another symbol of Jayson's vulnerability and weakness. Was he showing us again that there was still a big part of a small, helpless child in him? How possibly could a small child who was not even able to walk use the high-task tools of roller blades? Was the responsibility the doctors and nurses gave him by asking him to take over his treatment too overwhelming for him at his actual emotional developmental stage?

For the next two weeks his line did not work properly. I visited him every second to third day and witnessed his growing frustration and depression. One week I met him casually on a day that was not his dialysis day. He told me that he had to come to the unit an extra time because they had to remove extra fluid. "I drank too much. I'm not allowed to drink such a lot, but I did it anyway, I don't know why," was his explanation. Suddenly his rocket balls came to my mind, shooting at his future. Was he trying to drown his worries by drinking too much? Could this be considered a kind of chronic attempt at suicide because of his hopeless situation? However, aside from offering art therapy for catharsis by trying to help him to release his frustrations, there was nothing else I could do for him. As soon as I would try to address his feelings, he would shut down.

One day when I went looking for him – he had not been hooked up to his machine yet – I found him playing with one of the younger, severely handicapped children. It was so touching to see how careful and devoted teenage Jayson was by playing and fooling around with this small boy. Suddenly, the two children of his two collages (symbols for his own childlike soul?) came to my mind. Watching him play with this boy, I realized just how badly Jayson needed to be a child himself every once in a while, to be allowed to give up the burden of his disease. Since all the doctors and nurses and his social worker were working hard on his compliance and on his readiness to take over responsibility for his disease, I decided that my function should be different. I would allow him to be what he needs to be, rather than to address the same challenging things the others were doing.

On one day I came across him casually playing Nintendo in the storage room. He told me that he had to come to the hospital for several tests early in the morning and now he had to wait until the afternoon for his machine to be ready. Although it was not his day for art therapy, I suggested we have a session together sitting at a "real" table.

He quickly decided that he wanted to make another collage, one of cars (Figure 3.27: "Cars," collage by Jayson, 13 years). From his folder Jayson took out the saved car images and started, as usual, to cut and arrange the images carefully. Again, he was working meticulously and in silence. This time, he was more focused on closing as many gaps as possible, starting with the bigger and then filling in smaller images, even putting some upside down if the shape requested it. When he was done, Jayson did not want to give me any associations. He informed me that he still liked his very first collage best, adding that this one would be the last collage because he was tired of doing the same thing for too long, and that he would have to try something new next time. At the same time, he told me how much he enjoyed working at a real table. Together we explored possibilities for similar arrangements, but he did not want to come in earlier nor to stay longer after dialysis for art therapy. It was a decision that made perfect sense to me.

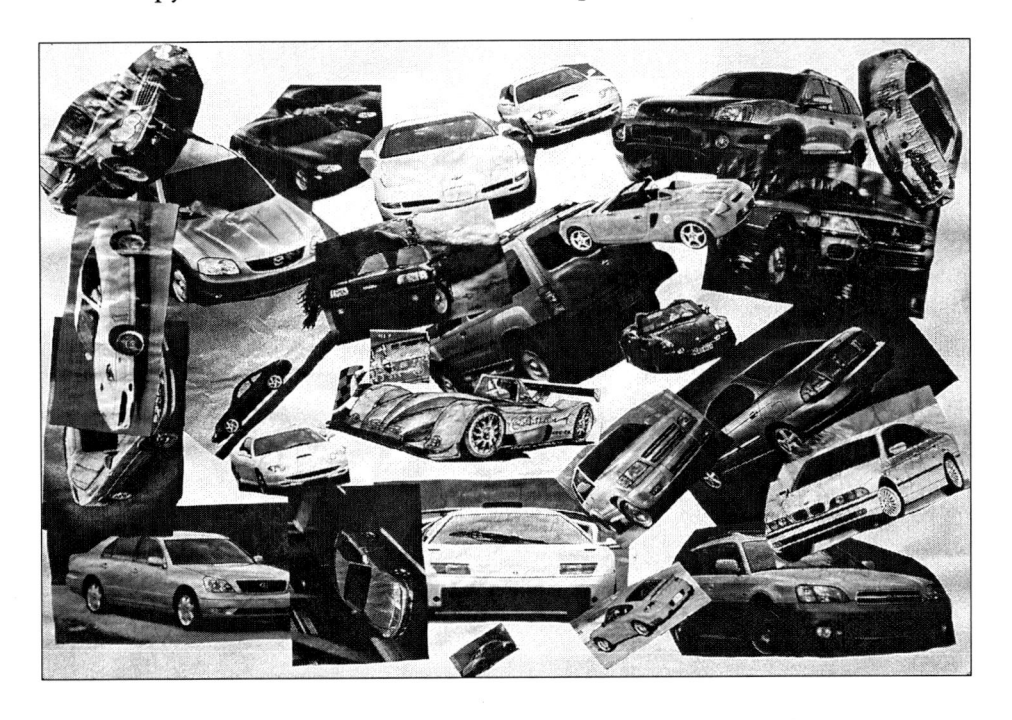

Figure 3.27. *Cars*, collage by Jayson, 13 years.

After taking a close look at this last collage, I found a small image of a red VW Beetle in the center, upside down, surrounded by strong sports cars. It reminded me of the ladybug he put in the center of his animal collage. However, this time he was not trying to leave the scene. Instead, he depicted himself in a helpless and hopeless situation, laying on his back, encircled by a lot of power. Was that how he perceived his actual situation?

When I met him for the following session, he was fine and ready to explore something new. Spontaneously, he suggested clay. For a long while he was just kneading and exploring the new material, while at the same time making plans of working after dialysis by sitting at a real table.

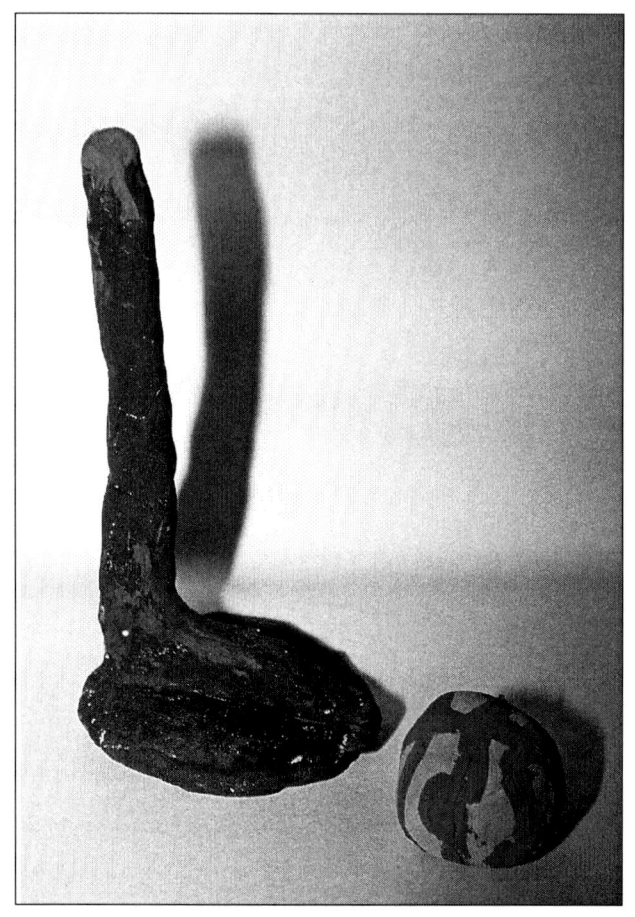

Figure 3.28. *In Honor of Hockey*, clay sculpture by Jayson, 13 years.

Then he started his actual piece: a baseball in all its details (Figure 3.28: "In Honor of Hockey," clay sculpture by Jayson, 13 years). He then decided to make another sculpture in "honor of Hockey" – a hockey stick sitting on top of a puck. For a long time, he was struggling with the stability of this long and fragile stick. Although he would not ask for help, he was able to accept my suggestion of using Popsicle sticks and toothpicks for stabilization. He finally succeeded and was very proud of it. He obviously was enjoying the new material, and was worked steadily through the whole session in silence. At the following session he finished the piece by painting it.

The repeated theme of sports seemed to be a means of extending his restricted world. Whereas in previous art pieces he used sports to release anger and aggression, on this day the associations were of sports trophies, about victories and awards. Did this represent his wish for being a "good boy," for being the winner of the situation? Was the struggle for stability of the stick his own struggle for stability?

At the following session he was fine, although he said his motivation for doing art was very low. Still, he agreed to have a session and decided to use paint (Figure 3.29: Untitled, watercolor by Jayson, 13 years).

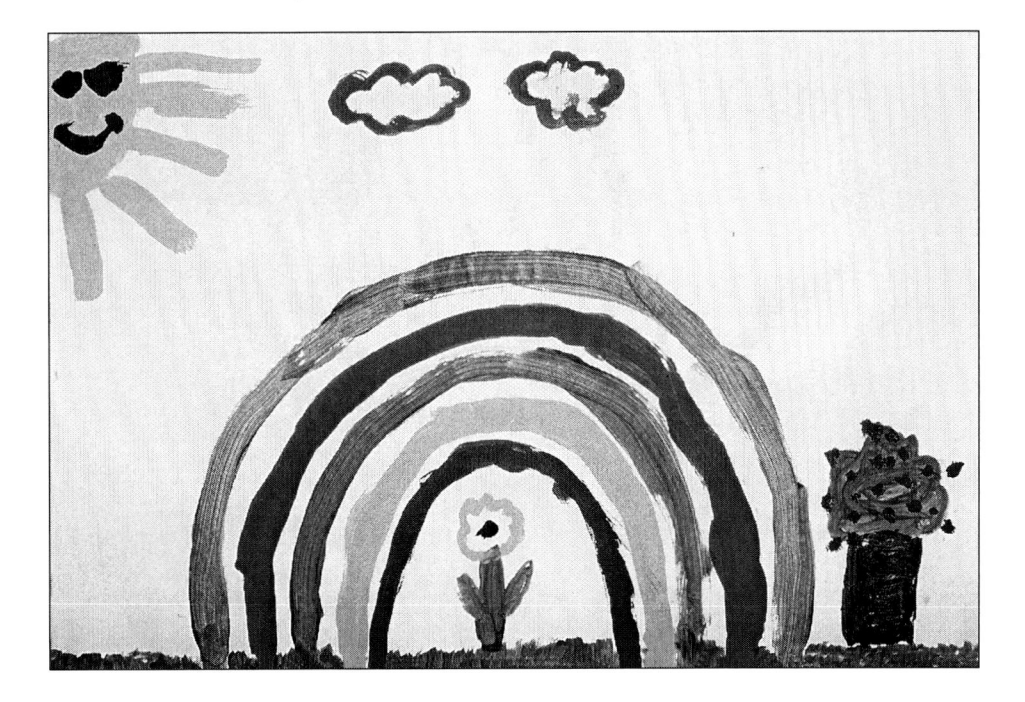

Figure 3.29. Untitled, watercolor by Jayson, 13 years.

Observing the way he was handling paint, I doubted that he felt comfortable with this material. Nevertheless he painted a flower under a heavy, colorful rainbow, a sun with critically-looking black eyes and a poor tree. He did not talk spontaneously for the full session, and did not disclose any associations at the end of it either.

This heavy rainbow reminded me again of the closed curtains of the stage. At the same time, it seemed to represent some sort of protective cave for this fragile lonely flower. In that sense it is striking how well-grounded the beams of the rainbow are, not allowing one single ant to penetrate. Whereas the tree with a short and thick trunk (similar to Jayson's own physical appearance) did not have any roots nor was it really grounded (there is a gap between the grass and the trunk). However, the sun with its black eyes was disturbing to me. I could sense the need for protection for this lonely vulnerable flower. Was the sun his transferential me, a scrutinizing authority? Was that how he felt about me as a representative for the whole medical team? The loneliness and isolation of the flower seemed to represent his own feelings of abandonment.

The week after he was fine. He was quick in making up his mind of what material to use: he chose clay. For a long time he did not have a theme, so he played with and explored the material by cutting, kneading, flattening, scratching and re-kneading it.

Finally, Jayson started to make some sort of construction with three clay sticks stabilized with a lot of Popsicle sticks (Figure 3.30: Untitled, clay sculpture by Jayson, 13 years). For a long time he struggled with the stability, but he would neither accept any help nor suggestions. I could feel a lot of ambivalence. On the one hand, he seemed to have some plans, which did not work out like he wanted, but on the other hand he did not feel the need to ask for help. There was also some sort of underlying boredom and lack of interest in whatever he was doing that day. His motivation was very low.

When he was done he did not want to give me any hint about the theme, or his associations. When I made a comment about my associations of a hockey goal, he frowned at me. With all the cracks and all the glue we used later to hold it together, I think it was unbearable for him to give this object any kind of title or meaning. It would show too much of his own fragility and threat of falling apart.

The following session I found him struggling with his homework. He told me that he did not have time to do art because he had to finish this piece of craft for school. I suggested finishing it as part of art therapy. He seemed to be more than happy to join in and explained the task. He had to make his own gold medal, thinking of himself as a winner of the Olympic games.

Together we explored the sport he would like to be the winner in and the way we could depict it, and so forth. We managed to finish a very nice, three-dimensional gold medal with laces to hang around his neck, thinking of him as an Olympic winner in hockey. He was very proud and happy about the result, and assured me that he would get a good mark for that piece.

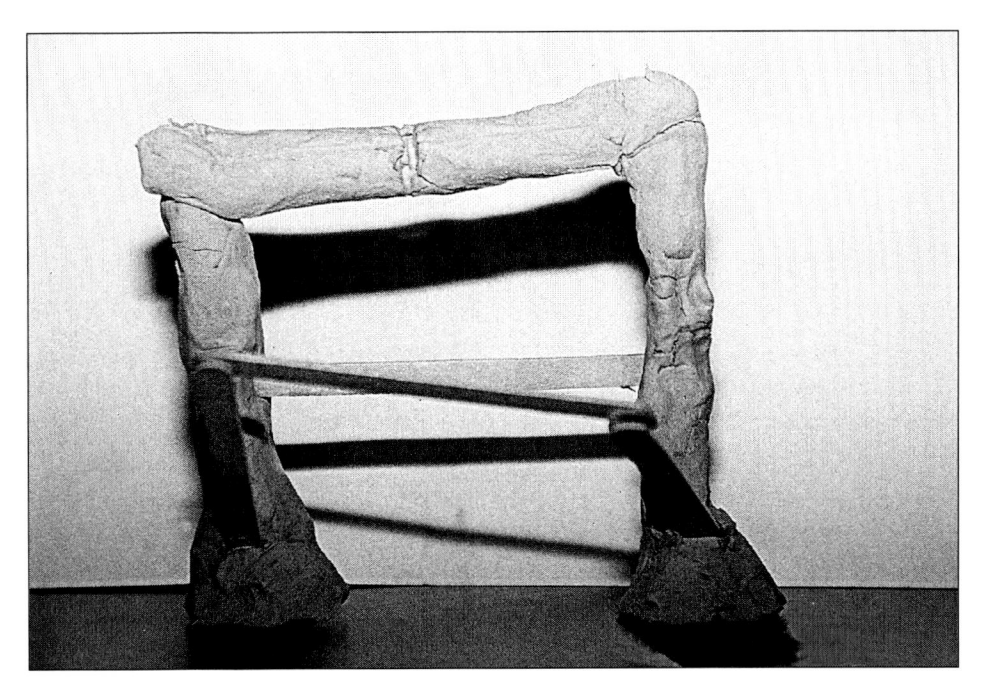

Figure 3.30. Untitled, clay sculpture by Jayson, 13 years.

During this session we were able to connect to each other very closely and to develop a well-balanced teamwork. In fact, we had never been so in tune with each other.

The following week he was ready to make art and wanted to use paint. Not having any idea of what to use as a subject, he asked for a directive. So I suggested a tree drawing, adding all the recommended assignments (Boland, 1977) (Figure 3.31: "My Tree," watercolor by Jayson, 13 years).

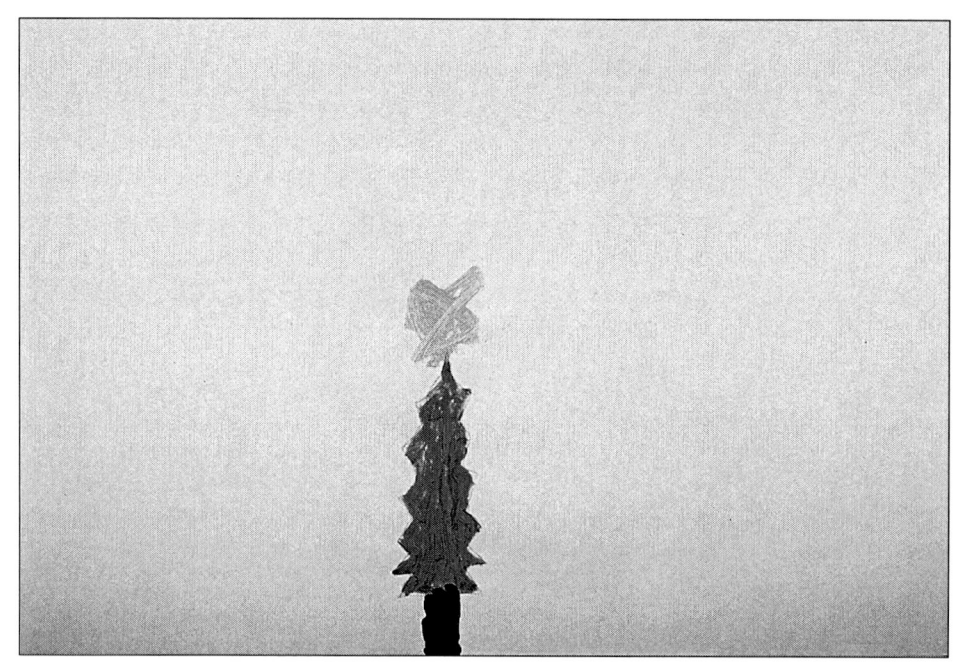

Figure 3.31. *My Tree*, watercolor by Jayson, 13 years.

He seemed to be interested in this theme and started to make a pencil drawing of a small pine in the middle of a huge piece of white paper. With the smallest brush he could find, he started to paint the tree and to turn it into a Christmas tree by adding a big star on the top. He was working with great concentration and did not make one single spontaneous comment. When I asked him what Christmas meant to him, he told me that he was Hindu and that they would not celebrate Christmas. However, they like the idea of exchanging gifts, and that was what they took over.

Suddenly he declared that he was done, and that he did not feel well. When the nurse came to measure his blood pressure, it was very low. Jayson had to lie down, and therefore, we were done with art therapy for today. Feeling better in this lying position, Jayson started to tell me about Hinduism, about the three temples in town and how they would celebrate their own kind of Christmas, with a lot of food and parties. It was the first time he shared all this information about his second culture with me.

I never got more associations about his tree-drawing, and I am still reluctant to use the usual score scale for interpretation for this purpose. Nonetheless, this picture definitively gives a sense of isolation and hopelessness. This small pine seemed to be overloaded with the huge golden star. At the same time, choosing the Christmas tree to represent his own tree to me was a similar symbol, like that of the rainbow and the colorful curtain, something to pretend happiness, where in reality sadness and desperation were hiding.

We missed several weeks of art therapy. First, because his line was not working properly and he therefore was immobilized. Second, when his line was working, he suffered from a terrible headache, due to intense hemodialysis. Again, he had drunk way too much, and they had to "dry him out," which resulted in a terrible headache due to a fast decrease in blood pressure. Third, another round of line problems as well as an inflammation and necrosis of the skin, which caused fever and fatigue.

I visited him every two to three days, hoping to be able to work with him. Although I usually stayed with him for a while, I felt useless and helpless. I got the feeling that, despite the strides we had made in our working relationship, we would never be able to reach a stage where Jayson had enough trust in me to make him feel secure.

For the last few weeks of his art therapy program Jayson worked on a longer project. He wanted to make a three-dimensional hand. So together we explored the possibilities of material: mold his own hand in clay and cast it in plaster; mold his hand by using plaster bandage; or, finally, cover a inflated surgical glove with papier-maché (Figure 3.32: "Michael Jackson's Glove," papier-maché sculpture by Jayson, 13 years).

He decided to go for the third technique. He invested two weeks in gluing several layers of cut newspaper and plain paper towels over the glove. He seemed to enjoy this artmaking process and was able not only to accept my help, but also to include me in his work process.

In the third week he wanted to add a last layer of paper towel in order to get a more neutral surface. After I had organized everything he did not accept any further help. I felt left out and useless, while he was working on his own without making any eye contact. He was tense and irritable. After a while, he let me know that he wanted to cut the entire thumb and all the fingertips. Answering my question "Why?" his only explanation was: to make it look like Michael Jackson's gloves.

After a while he started to tell me about the plan to move in with his uncle's family. He, his sister and his mother would move into his uncle's house and they would install everything needed for home dialysis. In two days, he and his mother would start their training in nightly home hemodialysis. I heard a strange ambivalence in his voice and asked him if he was looking forward to the upcoming change. His responses: "Yes" for moving in, "No" for the training in home hemodialysis because he was still hoping for another kidney transplant as a long-term solution. "But they don't want to test me again because they think I'm not ready for that, yet. It's a question of compliance, you know!" he told me in a way that did not allow me to ask more questions or to push this topic further.

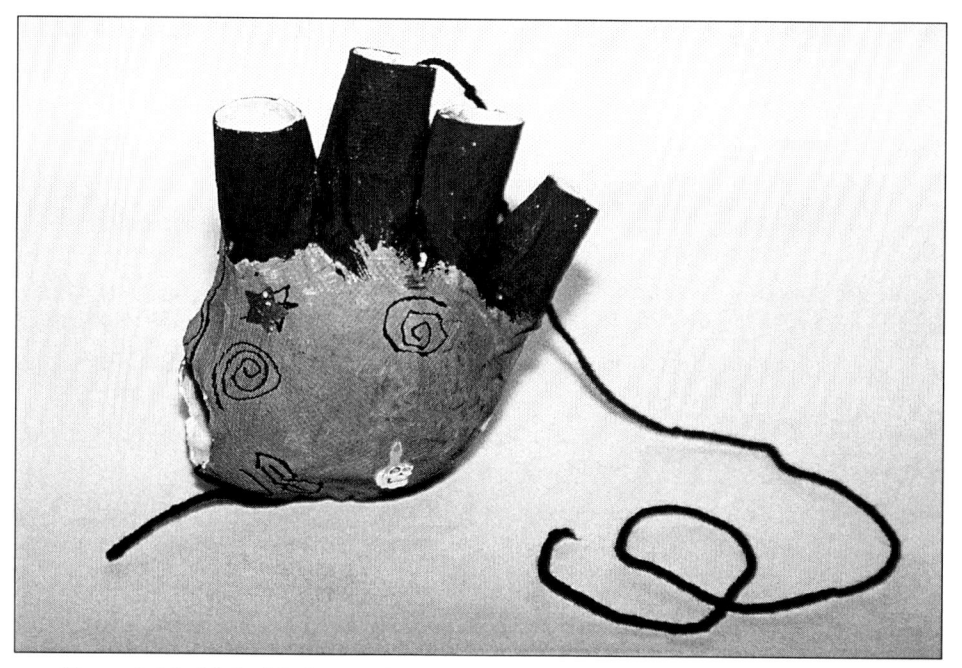

Figure 3.32. *Michael Jackson's Glove*, papier-maché sculpture by Jayson, 13 years.

I was wondering about his strange withdrawn behavior underlining his autonomy. Was it fear of becoming too dependent on me, when at the same time he was planning to gain independence from the hospital? And what was the metaphor of Michael Jackson's glove, his wish for independence and power similar to the role model of this pop star?

When I met Jayson the next time he was fine and wanted to pop the rubber glove in order to cut the thumb and the finger tips and to start to paint it. However, when he popped and removed the glove he realized that the papier maché layer was not thick enough to be stable. He was impatient and disappointed, and at the same time not motivated enough to add more paper. So he asked me if I could add a thick layer of paint. But I told him that paint would not stabilize the glove enough. So with some resistance he started to add more paper after cutting the thumb at its base and all the fingertips. We had to end this session earlier than planned because of a breakdown of his blood pressure with the usual consecutive symptoms.

While he was working he told me about the training he and his mother started and how difficult it was, how much there was to learn. Then he gave me a quick report about the installation work at his uncle's house. I thought it would be the right time to start termination with him. As soon as he and his mother would have finished their training, I told Jayson, he would not be coming to art therapy anymore. If he had any feelings, he sure did not show them. I could sense his growing anxiety and insecurity, without having any possible way to help him. As a result, I felt helpless myself.

I sensed his inner nervousness and restlessness, and some sort of ambivalence and underlying anxiety. At the same time, his glove without the thumb also reminded me of helplessness and powerlessness. What is the value of the powerful tool of a hand without its thumb?

At the following session he was fine, but not really motivated for art. At the same time, he wanted to paint and to finish his glove. In silence and with a stony face he started to cover the glove with blue paint. He was working very slowly, with very little motivation and interest in what he was doing. Again we had to stop this session earlier because of a breakdown of his blood pressure with consecutive symptoms.

As a result of his withdrawal and lack of enthusiasm, my subjective feeling was that I was left out, excluded or kicked out of a working program. Did I pick up his anxiety of being kicked out and abandoned by the hospital once he would have finished his training in home dialysis? The closer the date of the moving came, the bigger his ambivalence, his restlessness and nervousness grew.

Again we lost another week of art therapy because of symptoms due to too-low blood pressure during intense hemodialysis.

When I met him the next time he looked awful, with dark rings under his eyes. Nevertheless he wanted to finish his glove. Very slowly and in total silence he painted the amputated fingers in black. But soon he had to give up again because of dizziness and nausea due to low blood pressure. Again we had to stop the session earlier.

That day I was a little bit too early and was able to observe mother and son during their training in hemodialysis. Suddenly I had the feeling that Jayson's physical tendency to faint was another sign of his emotional wish to give up. Everything was just too much for him. I realized that my helplessness and hopelessness was my projective identification with Jayson's desperation. He seemed to be scared of losing the secure base of the hospital, one that he had learned to trust in over the years, and he was not able to trust himself and his mother to take its place.

At the last session he definitely wanted to finish his glove. After a long and critical look at it, he asked for the box with stickers. But first he wrote his full name with black markers onto the palm and the back of the glove. Very carefully and slowly he then chose the stickers and placed them – a skull with a candle on top, three blue stars, a soccer ball, a bat and a red sports car with the printing "super kid." He still did not seem to be satisfied and tried several ways to make the glove stand on a surface or to hang it. Finally, he asked for a string with which to hang it. His final look was one of satisfaction and pride. He made it!

During this session his machine sounded an alarm several times. With a dramatic, but proud gesture he manipulated the machine, showing me how autonomous he was now in controlling his dialysis. I paid him a big compliment. He suddenly seemed to gain some self-confidence.

Although he wanted, as his last art project, to make a dream catcher for his new room at his uncle's house, I could not convince him to do any art for these last two weeks. He didn't have any physical symptoms, but he was either too nervous and restless or too tired. Soon his family would move into their new home. Then he would get his own hemodialysis machine installed in his new bedroom. I could understand that he was going through too much of a change to be able to concentrate on art. Whenever I met him, he told me how things were going.

During his very last week his final night training in hemodialysis was planned. He and his mother had to sleep at the hemodialysis unit with a nurse, in order to prove that they were able to deal with the machine on their own. I was hoping to join them for one or two evenings to make a dream catcher with Jayson, but he showed a very avoidant behavior, very much supported by his mother.

I had a hard time trying to organize a final session in order to get a last opportunity to meet him and to review the last nine months of art therapy together. But when I did he was looser and seemed to be happier and more secure. We had a nice final chat during which he told me about his first week of experience with nightly home hemodialysis, and how better his blood pressure was and how healthier he would feel in general. I had the feeling he was telling me the truth. He made his first jump into more independence from the hospital.

He summarized his experience in art therapy – in general, he enjoyed it and would join in again, maybe by doing more craft than art. Art therapy for him was helpful in distracting him and in helping him to free his mind because he did not have to think all the time about his disease and about being compliant. It was the place where he had some freedom, and where there were no rebukes.

SUMMARY

Thirteen-year-old Jayson was withdrawn and not very talkative. For the whole duration of nine months treatment, he performed a defiant resistance, apparently keeping me in safe distance from him. Although apparently he was not into art, he never quit art therapy spontaneously. This insecure attachment dynamic perhaps reflected his attachment with his mother. He carefully tried to hide any kind of emotions, positive and/or negative. Although appearing emotionally flat, there was a deep underlying sadness rooting in anger and frustration. That was most likely the way he had to deal with his emotions around his physical illness, and around his father's death as well. In his family there was no place for grief and mourning losses. He often used art in a catharctic way. His artwork mainly reflected his feelings of frustration and anger, of powerlessness and hopelessness, and of being overwhelmed. During the session with him I often felt left out, like sitting in front of a stage with closed curtains, knowing that there was a drama playing behind them, but not being allowed to participate. I wonder if it was like he felt in life.

6. Katja, Female, 12 Years

Description of the Client

Katja is a twelve-year-old Asian girl. Her round face with full cheeks was caused by her chronic steroid medication. Otherwise, she was of short stature with a very fragile appearance. Physically she seemed to just be entering puberty since she had very little in the way of secondary female features.

From the very beginning she exhibited an open, friendly but extremely shy, withdrawn behavior. Initially, she made only very short eye contact. She did not talk directly to me, but asked for her child life specialist to be present and to transmit her whispered answers to my questions. Only after two sessions did Katja trust me enough to allow her child life specialist to leave the session for short periods of time. At the beginning she never talked spontaneously, but replied to my questions with whispered, as-short-as-possible answers. It took a few weeks to have a spontaneous conversation. She obviously had very low self-esteem and self-confidence.

Usually she was of even mood and had good impulse control. Because of her concrete way of thinking, she had great difficulties in verbalizing feelings. She would, though, express them non-verbally through body language and in her art.

She loved doing art and crafts, and was therefore open to exploring new techniques despite her huge insecurity and low self-confidence. Often I had to lead her hands or make an outline drawing for her because she was almost blocked by a fear of failure.

Social History

Katja was the middle of three children, and had a fourteen-year-old sister and a six-year-old brother. Both parents were of Vietnamese origin. Her father had immigrated twenty years earlier, her mother seventeen years ago. Her mother owned a cosmetic salon. Her father had worked for the same company as a production supervisor for the past seventeen years. At the job, he enjoyed a good reputation and immense support from his employers – a support particularly valued because of the time he needed to take off work in order to bring Katja to dialysis appointments three times a week. In general, it was the father who seemed to be much more engaged and involved in Katja's care. He was also the most competent person in terms of giving information about his daughter's state of health. Katja's mother was a nice, but more superficial type of person, seemingly more engaged by caring for her daughter's appearance (clothing, hairstyle, nail polish, etc.), which Katja appeared to be proud of. But her real attachment was more with her father.

Katja was a grade seven student with poor academic results. Due to her disease, she missed a lot of school. For the two days per week she was off dialysis, she attended public school. During dialysis three times a week, the hospital teacher worked with her. In addition, she had home teaching over the weekends. With this program there was little time left for social activities. Katja never talked a lot about friendships. Although she was well-embedded in her supportive family, she did not have a lot of peer contact apart from what took place at public school. Adding to her isolation was the fact she never was able to attend school trips or take part in other social activities outside of her familial circle.

In general, the three siblings seemed to have a healthy relationship, and loved one another. But because of her fragility, Katja was often overwhelmed by the more straightforward personalities of her two siblings.

Medical History

Up until one year ago, when Katja's disease started, she was a totally healthy and easy child. Compared to her more robust sister, she was shy and fragile and, therefore, a more devoted child. At that time she was still a good student.

Three months before I met her, she became severely ill, vomited and lost consciousness. She had to be admitted to the hospital by ambulance. The doctors diagnosed an end-stage renal failure and a juvenile diabetes mellitus caused by a complex rheumatologic disease. Typical for this disease are circulating auto-antibodies, which attack a person's kidneys, lungs, brain and, in Katja's case, pancreas tissue. The inflammation caused by the auto-antibodies destroys these tissues. Katja was immediately put on high-dose steroids and intense immunosuppression. But her kidneys and her pancreas did not recover, and there was damage to her brain as well. She needed kidney replacement therapy, and was insulin-dependent. She also developed low-grade seizure activity, which resulted in two major seizures.

In summary, for three months Katja was in and out of the intensive care unit, and went through a huge disfigurative change in her appearance due to the medication. She suffered all the possible complications listed in a medical textbook in relation to her disease, including gastrointestinal bleeding and skin problems.

Since the onset of her disease, she had been on regular hemodialysis. As long as the activity of her rheumatologic disease was not under optimal control, kidney transplantation was not an option. Katja was always cooperative and showed a good compliance in her treatment, including her insulin regulation.

Art Therapy Process and Artwork

We started the art therapy program, which lasted for 38 sessions, three months after the sudden onset of her disease. She was referred to me by her social worker, who thought art therapy might help with Katja's low self-esteem and self-confidence. The shy and fragile child had been thrown back in her developmental stage by the severe disease.

For our first session she refused to meet me on her own, but asked that her child life specialist, Linda, be present. Making only brief eye contact, Katja did not talk to me directly. Rather, she made Linda answer my questions. Katja definitely showed an interest in the art material I introduced and demonstrated to her. To bridge the initial hesitation I suggested to Katja that she decorate the cover of her personal folder, to which she agreed. But when it came to make a decision about what technique to use, a long and painful silence developed. Eventually, Linda made a suggestion to cut the letters of Katja's name out of colored paper and glue them onto the cover. This was my first experience with a typical Katja reaction. Whenever she encountered a new situation, she would declare her incapability and have somebody else make the first example. So I ended up cutting the letters for Katja according to her detailed instructions about the type of letter and color of paper. However, those detailed instructions, even though they were just whispers, marked the first time she directly communicated with me. Soon she was using the glue and sticking the letters onto the cover herself. Suddenly she appeared totally enthusiastic about the process. As I learned later, she loved glue – lots of glue!

For the following session Katja wanted to have Linda with her again. As Linda and I had discussed after the previous session, she was to be present at the beginning of the second session, and then leave us after a while, explaining to Katja that she would have to look after other children as well. On this day, Katja had chosen to work in clay but was not able to do anything. For a long time she would only knead and roll the clay, enjoying the touch of its moist stickiness and doing so in silence. After a long while she whispered that she did not know what to make. I suggested she make different animals that represented her family members. After a while she decided to make a Teddy bear for herself, but quickly added that she did not know how to do it. Step by step I showed her how to roll balls for head and trunk, and rolls for the limbs. She made me put the figure together, following very attentively each of my movements. Eventually we made two Teddy bears, one standing and one sitting. After a short contemplation she asked in a very low voice if she was allowed to add something to the standing bear. Very slowly and carefully she rolled a tiny apple and put it into the bear's paws. A long eye contact showing pride asked for acknowledgment. I was so proud of her – it was her very first spontaneous and independent action with me.

She was waiting for me without Linda at the following session. Not only did she no longer need the support of the child life specialist, Katja had gained enough trust with me to let me know her plans for today. First, make another object in clay; then paint her Teddy bears. Though she spoke in a low voice, which reflected her insecurity, and spent many minutes silently kneading and rolling the clay, she did eventually offer a suggestion of what to make: a pumpkin with a happy face (Figure 3.33: "Happy Pumpkins," clay sculpture by Katja, 12 years).

Obviously she was looking for something she could make on her own with a shape she had already learned. Nevertheless, she needed a fair bit of encouragement. For the whole session she did not talk spontaneously, apart from asking for help. Still, she seemed to enjoy the opportunity to explore more autonomy by using the basic shape of the ball, and ended up making two pumpkin heads. Finally, she was satisfied with the result and declared that she wanted to paint both pumpkin faces next time when they were dry. To finish the session she painted her Teddy bears, asking for help with the handling of the paint. After a long, satisfied look – one that had a measure of pride – she asked in an even lower voice than usual: "May I take them home today? I like them so much!" I agreed, telling her that she was allowed to take home her clay sculptures (since I was lacking of storage space). However, I also reminded her that her picture and drawings would have to stay in her folder with me until the end of the program. At the same time I assured her that she was – and would remain – the owner of her art. I had the feeling she needed to take it home as a reward for her breakthrough out of withdrawal.

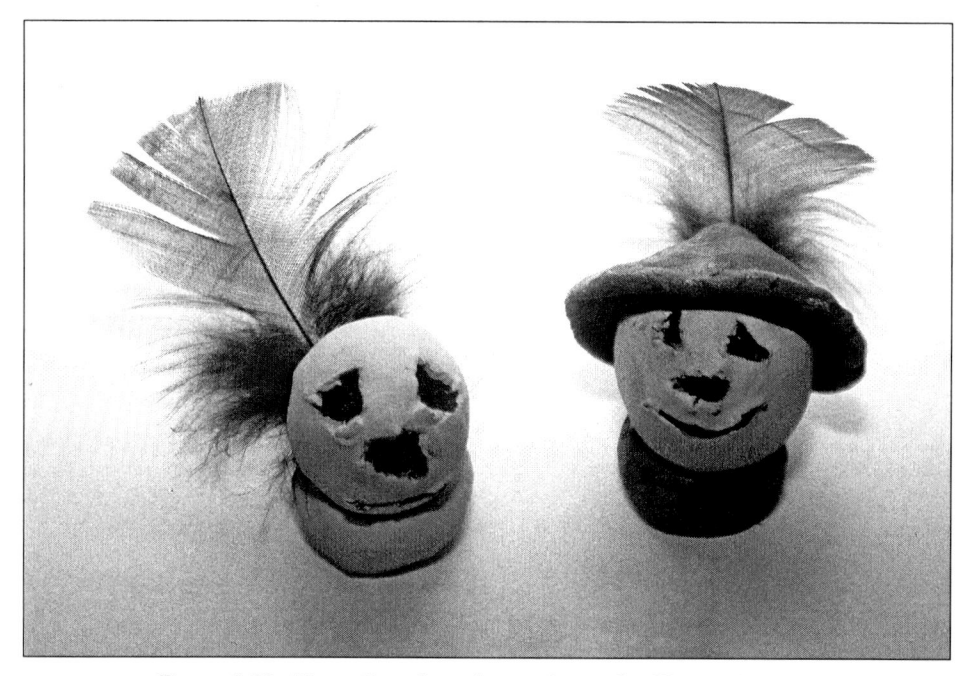

Figure 3.33. *Happy Pumpkins*, clay sculpture by Katja, 12 years.

At this point the art therapy program had to be interrupted due to Katja's severe gastrointestinal bleeding, which made intensive care necessary. I visited her several times as an inpatient, just to spend some time with her. Although we did not talk a lot, these visits seemed to be important for our relationship, providing continuity. When I met her for the following session, she was an outpatient again and she was waiting for me. First she wanted to paint her pumpkin faces, and then her plan was to start a new clay object. She decided to make a bee (Figure 3.34: "Bees," clay sculpture with box by Katja, 12 years).

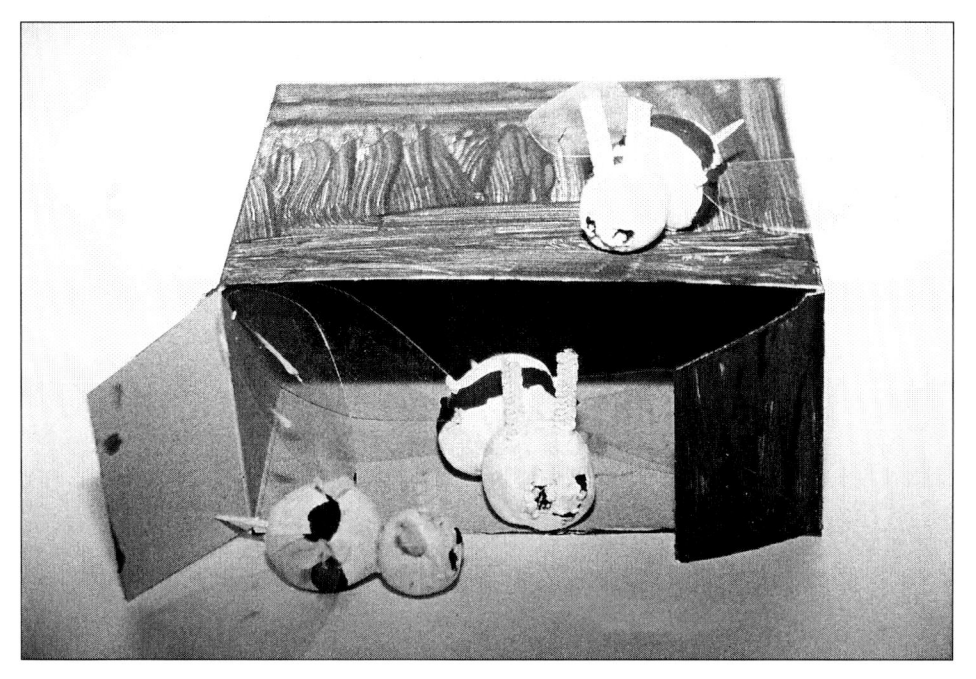

Figure 3.34. *Bee Family*, clay sculpture by Katja, 12 years.

She started right away to make different sizes of balls for the body and head. Then she asked for help in sticking them together. I showed her the trick with the toothpicks. But the toothpick was a little too long and could be seen on the rear end of the bee. At first she wanted to cut the toothpick; then she remembered that bees sting – and the toothpick could be the bee's stinger. Finally she asked for help with the wings, which we made out of plastic. After she finished the first bee, adding a smiling face, she immediately wanted to make a whole family. It was amazing to watch her – how with each bee she gained more security and, therefore, more autonomy. While she was working she told me that she liked bees because they looked like cute little flying bears, and because she liked honey. I wondered how that would match with her diabetes diet. When she had a final look at her bees she discovered that the baby bee had the longest stinger. "In fact all of them have very long stings," was her comment. And for the first time in a louder voice, she added: "But they need them to defend themselves, especially the baby bee." I was surprised to hear her full voice for the first time and was wondering if that was her reflection of her family's need for protection after last months' heavy attacks.

She spent the next session painting the bees, taking extra care to paint the stingers in ardent red. When she was done she wanted to make a beehive from a cardboard box, where her bees could get shelter. At the end of the session she had a final, satisfied look at her bee family in front of its hive. "I like them. I would like to take them home as soon as possible." And then she told me about a shelf that she had prepared at home. It would exhibit all her clay sculptures, including the Teddy bears and pumpkin faces that were already there. The wish to take her work home in combination with her typical way of involving me in a very characteristic, well-balanced teamwork illustrated that she trusted me and would find ways to connect with me.

Two days later, after I finished work with another child, she made a signal for me to join her. "I can't wait to take my bees home," she explained. Although it was not a day for her session, she asked me to help wrap her bee family in order to take it home. Before wrapping each single bee carefully in tissue paper and embedding it into the hive, she polished the wings with almost passionate dedication. A final contemplation of the stingers, especially of baby bee's stinger, was accompanied by admiration: "Isn't she cute, so small, so friendly looking but nevertheless so valiant." Suddenly I sensed a big ambivalence: on the one hand I had the feeling Katja was identifying with the baby bee; on the other hand the baby bee had qualities that were different than her own. I could sense her high admiration and respect for the baby bee. Then we closed the hive. "Now they are safe," was her comment. She gave me a big happy smile. That was the moment for me to tell her how proud I was of her because she had developed, in just a few weeks, a wonderful autonomy.

The week after I was very surprised to find the tight-closed beehive in the cupboard for art and crafts. I asked Katja if she forgot to take it home last time. Avoiding eye contact, she mumbled a strange excuse: she said she didn't have enough space in her bag. But when I later found the hive hidden in an even remoter corner of the cupboard, I began wondering if her admiration for these brave animals had turned into fear – that they could now be a threat. I also started to wonder whether the stinger of these animals represented her desire for more valiant bearing, or rather her own unconscious anger and aggression, now threatening her. Therefore, it was less the bee family being saved (as she told me with a big smile of relief), but rather herself being saved of the bees.

At the following session she looked pale and very tired. Nevertheless, she wanted to do art. Giving me a pencil, she asked if I could draw a dog for her. I told her that I would draw a dog on a separate piece of paper by following her detailed description about size, features and position; and then she could copy it. But today she seemed to be too weak. So I decided to let her color my drawing. Halfway through we had to stop the session. In a very low voice and with tears in her eyes, she suddenly told me she felt sick, and asked me to call her nurse. She had a very low blood pressure and had to be laid back to avoid shock symptoms.

Two days later – I had just finished cleaning up from a session with another child – I found Katja's father looking for any kind of entertainment for her. She had to lie flat because her line was not working – and Linda had no time for her. So she was in a very bad mood. I offered to make up her last session, which had to be terminated too soon. But it was difficult to find something to do with her given that she was laying flat. Finally, I suggested that we do something with pipe cleaners, which were easy to bend and to work with even when not sitting at a table. She liked the idea and decided to make a bird (Figure 3.35: "Bird," pipe cleaner object by Katja, 12 years). But, as happened at the beginning of the program, she quickly added in a low voice that she was not capable of making one. In fact, she had no idea how to start. Was it the new material, her prostrate position or the setback of her physical condition that caused this regression?

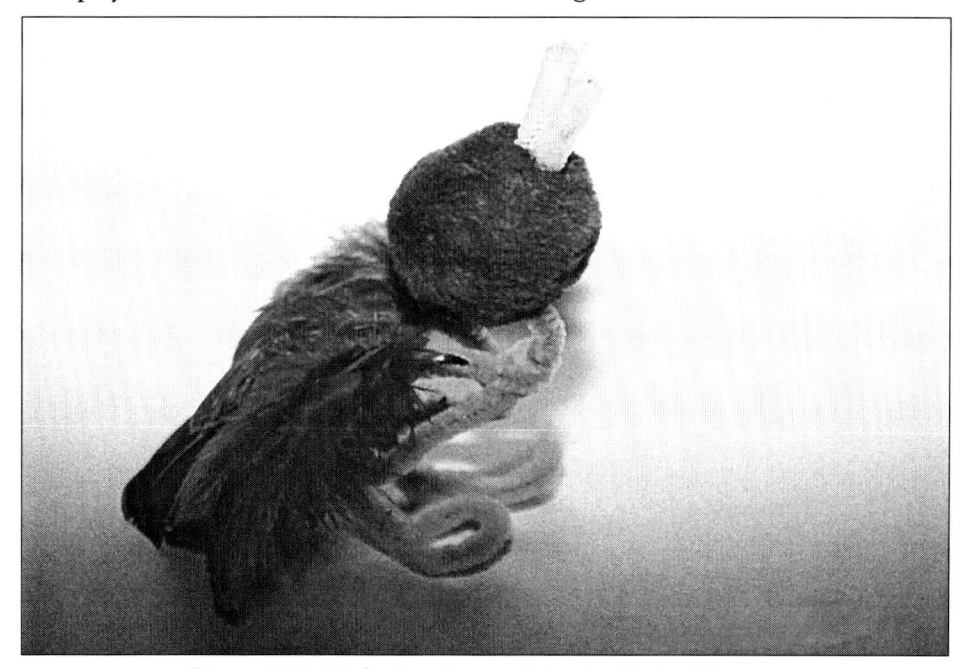

Figure 3.35. *Bird*, pipe-cleaner object by Katja, 12 years.

Following her detailed description of the bird she had in mind, I showed her how to make it, including a woolen ball for the head and feathers for the wings. She was totally happy with her bird and asked: "Will it be dry to take home for the next session? And can we make more next time?" She seemed to be restored again.

At the following session she had recovered, and was waiting for me. After taking a brief satisfied look at her bird, she decided to work in clay and make another Teddy bear (Figure 3.36: "Teddy Bear," clay sculpture by Katja, 12 years).

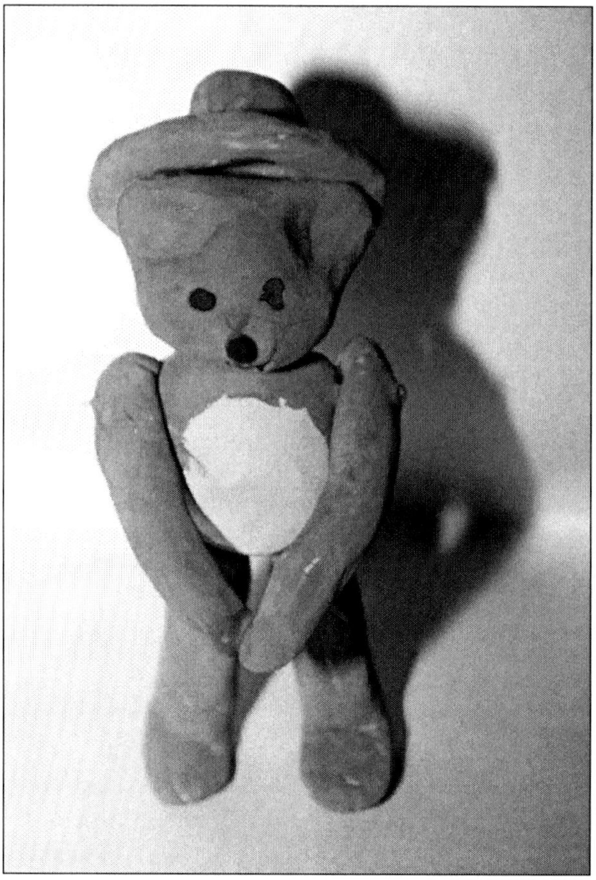

Figure 3.36. *Teddy Bear*, clay sculpture by Katja, 12 years.

For a while she did not know how to start and wanted me to make the bear for her. But after a while she seemed to remember how and started to make different sizes of balls and rolls, and asked only for help in sticking them together with toothpicks. She also asked for help with the hat. Although she had already made a Chinese hat for her pumpkin face, she pretended not to know how to make it. I felt reluctant, but then I remembered the function of a hat: beside decoration, a hat protected a person against rain or sun. While making the desired hat, I wondered if she, in her vulnerability, was symbolically asking for protection.

At the following session she painted her Teddy bear. Then she had another look at her pipe-cleaner bird. Quickly she decided that it needed a cage in which to take shelter (Figure 3.37: "Bird's Cage," Popsicle stick object by Katja, 12 years).

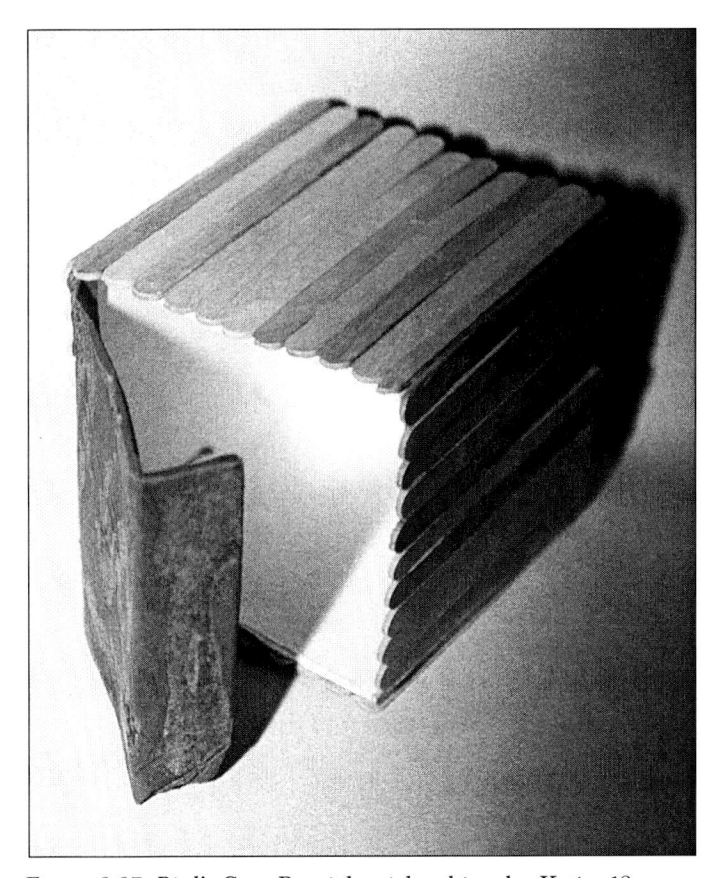

Figure 3.37. *Bird's Cage*, Popsicle sticks object by Katja, 12 years.

Using a cardboard box as a base, she chose to use Popsicle sticks and tissue paper. While she was working on the bird's house, she started to tell me about her house, which was made of red bricks, and about who was with her. It was the first time she started to talk spontaneously, beyond simple technical comments. In a somewhat uninvolved way, like a neutral external observer, she described her family, including her aunt and little niece who lived in the same house. I was surprised about the lack of emotional involvement, and wondered if she felt left out.

Another striking thing was her need to have her figures wear hats or to build shelters for them. To me the hats and shelters were metaphors for her own need for protection, and therefore a reflection of her own vulnerability.

Finally, I was surprised by the amount of glue she used in order to stick the Popsicle sticks. There was glue everywhere; she was almost drowning in glue. Similar to her work in clay, she seemed to enjoy the moist stickiness of the glue. I had the association of a very young child in an early developmental stage, who needed to physically explore his environment. Was that another sign of the regression she suffered as a result of her extremely difficult time over the last few months? Or was she making up for a missed developmental step of her own early childhood?

At the following session she seemed to be very tired. Nevertheless, she wanted to make a collage. Last time I had mentioned a collage technique that used colored tissue paper while we were using the same approach with the cage's door. Immediately she wanted to know more about it.

She knew exactly the composition of the picture: a Christmas tree and a bird underneath (Figure 3.38: "Christmas Tree," collage by Katja, 12 years). As with every new situation, she declared that she was not able to make the drawing, and that I had to make it for her. This time her statement was made in a firm voice. For a while I tried to convince her that she should at least try to do it. But more and more she developed an almost stubborn defiance. To stop from losing her overall interest, I decided to make the outline drawing according to her precise description of type, size and position of the bird and tree. Happily, she started to tear tissue paper and glue it onto the outline drawing, again using a huge amount of glue. Her major concern was to spare the pencil marks. Carefully she filled in the spaces with colored tissue paper, adding layer after layer. For the whole time she worked with great concentration and in absolute silence.

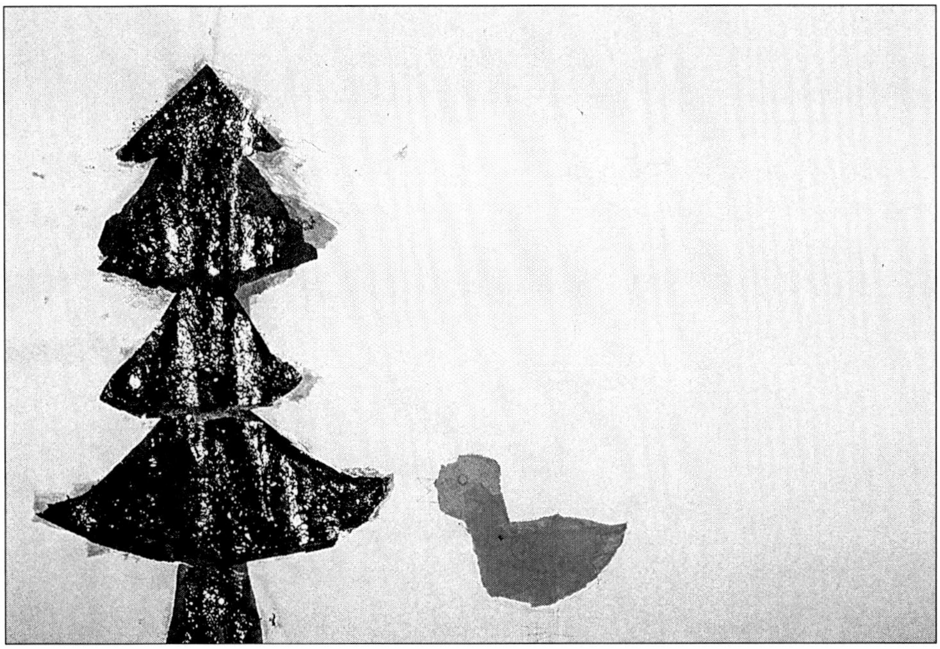

Figure 3.38. *Christmas Tree*, collage by Katja, 12 years.

It took her three sessions to finish this piece. The longer she worked on it, the more security she gained. I had the feeling she needed the security of the outline drawing to contain her own weak self; and now she gained security by filling in her projected self into this "container." She had gained so much security it seemed that she felt safe enough to engage me in another conversation while she worked. This time the theme was school, and how often she had to miss it. But she was always there for the art class, and she loved this class. She continued to tell me about all the techniques they were learning. This time I could sense a healthy, positive emotional involvement in her conversation. I was especially surprised by her enthusiasm about the sketching at school, whereas with me she was very reluctant about making her own drawing. This confirmed my hypothesis about her need for containment to develop and nurture her security and self-confidence.

At the following session she was almost high-spirited and declared that she wanted to work in clay again (Figure 3.39: "Snowman," clay sculpture by Katja, 12 years).

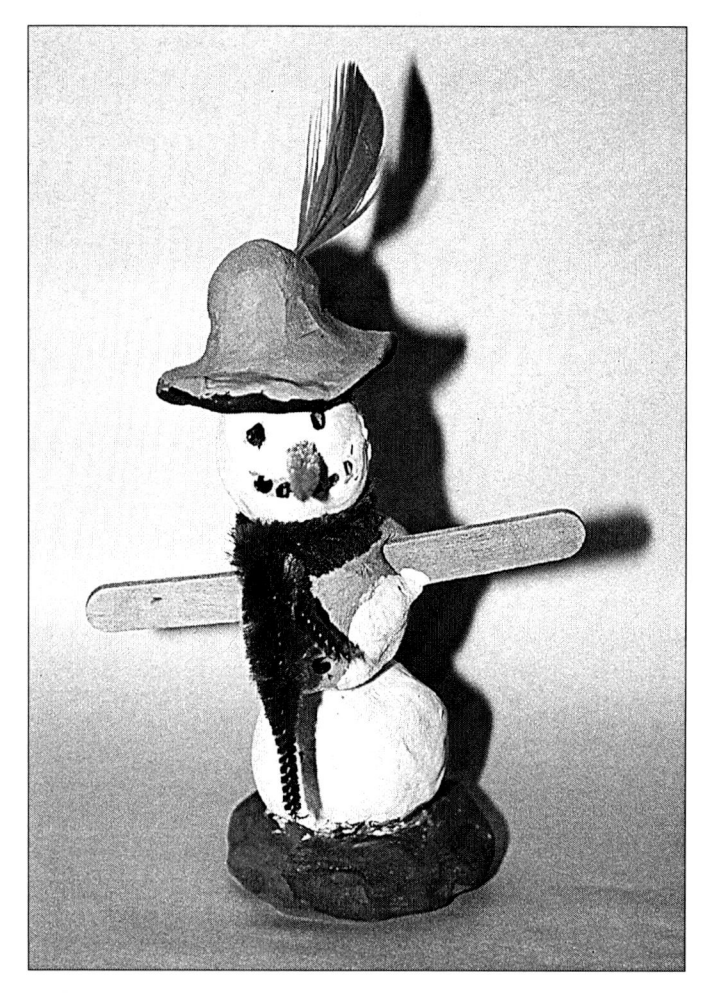

Figure 3.39. *Snowman*, clay sculpture by Katja, 12 years.

She decided to make a snowman since it was snowing outside. Immediately she added that she did not know how to make one. Before I could say something, her neighbor (Jayson, 13 years) turned around and said "You girls are all weird. Just take three balls, one bigger than the other, the smallest for the head and the biggest for the bottom." For a short moment they continued teasing each other in a funny and flirtatious way, behavior I had not observed before. Then Jayson turned back and did not pay attention to her anymore. Showing a surprising autonomy she followed the advice and finished the snowman, using a pipe cleaner for the nose and scarf. With a final look she announced that she would paint it next time, adding that she wanted to put it under the Christmas tree at home.

In order to fulfill her wish, we had to fit in an additional session to paint the snowman. I did not mind because it would mean that we could make up for some of the missed sessions when she was feeling sick. It took her a long time to mix the brown, but she seemed to enjoy the mixing part of this "dirt-like" material. Unfortunately, we had to interrupt this session earlier than planned due to her medical conditions. What's more, she never wanted to finish the snowman and abandoned him at the end of the program. With this snowman she ended the phase of exploration in clay for the rest of the program.

The following session, Katja was accompanied by her sister Julie. I had a hard time convincing Julie that she should leave us alone for one hour. When we were finally on our own, Katja quickly decided that she would finish her Christmas tree collage, the one in which the bird was left unfinished. I was surprised how secure she was in the tearing of the paper, and the gluing of it. We were interrupted twice by Julie, who could not bear to be excluded. The first time Katja showed Julie her collage with pride, obviously enjoying the admiration of her bigger sister. But when Julie asked if she could join us because she liked this technique, Katja was faster than I was in answering: "No, that's my time. That's my special therapy." I was very surprised. At the second interruption Julie tried to correct Katja, telling her that ducks had to be yellow, not orange. Katja's immediate answer was: "This is not just a duck. It is a special bird, and special birds have any colors." Her sister definitively withdrew. Again I was surprised by the security Katja had developed which led to this spirited defense of her own art. I tried to find out a little bit more about Katja's special bird. But suddenly there was nothing special anymore. As usual Katja did not want to give her associations to the final image. I made a comment about the firmness Katja had showed in defending her rights and position with her sister – that was special for me, and I was proud of her. When she was done with collaging the bird, she felt that the picture was complete, although the right side of the paper was still empty, and the bird still had very weak legs and beak. I wondered if the almost invisible thin legs and beak of the bird were mirroring her own weakness. Finally, I wondered about the big empty space to the right half of the paper: Did this empty space reflect her struggle with the unpredictability of her future?

For the next session she decided to explore a new technique. She wanted to learn about oil pastels because her class was using them in

138 *Art Therapy with Chronic Physically Ill Adolescents*

art class, and she had to miss that session at her school. She asked me to make a drawing of a person for her since she said she was incapable of drawing one. As I discussed with my supervisor, I would serve her as "auxiliary ego" and help her to develop strength by offering her the containment she needed. Without objections, I started to draw, according to the detailed description of the girl she had in mind (Figure 3.40: "A Sitting Girl," oil pastels by Katja, 12 years).

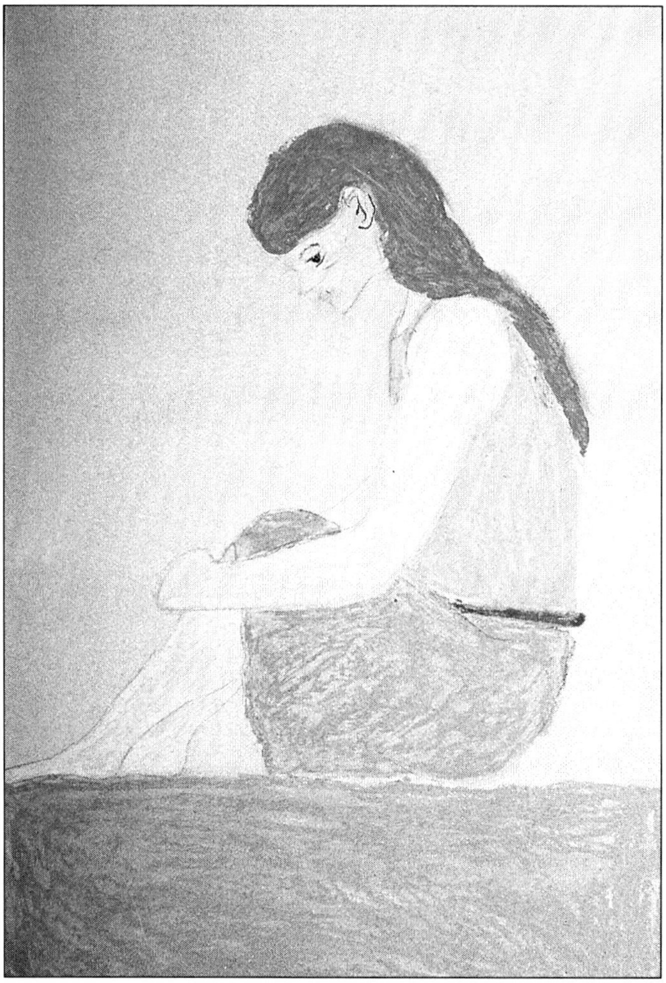

Figure 3.40. *A Sitting Girl,* oil pastels by Katja, 12 years.

Whatever Katja told me about the girl (view, position, gesture, body and facial features, etc.) I put to paper. She was very satisfied with the result and started right away to color with oil pastels. While she was working, she told me about a huge box of oil pastels she got for Christmas. But because she did not know how to use them, Julie was using them. Now she was looking forward to asking for them back, since she was the legal owner. Together we had a final look at the picture. Although she was satisfied with the result, she did not want to give me any associations. I did not insist because I thought that there was too much of it that was from my own hand. Nevertheless I was touched by the underlined sadness in the position of that girl, looking back and down to the "past" corner of the image.

The following session she was impatiently waiting for me because she had a new picture in mind: a forest in oil pastels (Plate 7: "My White Rabbit," oil pastel by Katja, 12 years, p. 48).

For a while we discussed different types of trees, and I showed her how to make them in oil pastel onto a separate piece of paper. Then she started to make a bright blue sky. As usual, she took green and brown and started to copy my trees onto her paper. I was thrilled by this big progress, and I paid her a compliment. When she was done with the forest she started to contemplate the big empty space in the foreground. In a lower voice she expressed her wish for a running rabbit, but did not know how to make it. She asked me for an outline drawing. It was obvious that after all the exploring of new ground she needed containment and had to move back to a secure base. I drew the rabbit, which she colored in white. The figure of the white rabbit re-emerged in several of her pictures later on. I had the feeling she was identifying herself with it and, therefore, I was happy to see her move towards the "future" part of the picture.

For several weeks she worked in oil pastel, following the same pattern of having me make outline drawings for her. Her rheumatologic disease seemed to be more active again. She often suffered from red, swollen eyes, swollen face and general fatigue. Knowing that her disease could compromise her central nervous system, I wondered about the involvement of her eyes in the autoimmune process (e.g., uveitis, iridocyclitis, etc.). Unfortunately, I could not get any conclusive answer from either the nurses or the doctors. Trusting my own medical experience, I noticed how reduced in strength she was; and therefore, how regressive her behavior. According to her need I tried to function as her "auxiliary ego" by having her give me as precise instruction as possible for the requested outline drawings. I wanted the picture to mirror her as much as possible. The themes were mostly animals: a sitting cat licking its fur, a sitting white rabbit, a sitting pink pig, and so on. All animals were depicted in profile, heading towards the right (future related) side of the paper. As usual she refused to give me any associations in regard to the pictures. I had the feeling she was in a kind of resting stage in her development. She needed to be – and enjoyed being – contained by me. My hypothesis was confirmed when she made a comment about the white rabbit needing a rest. While she was coloring the sitting rabbit image, she explained: "This is my white rabbit running through my forest in my previous picture. You remember? He has to sit and have a rest for a while."

One day I found her again as an in-patient. She had to be hospitalized due to a major seizure and needed iv-medication. From Linda I learned that she was very depressed. So when I met her I was not surprised by her choice of oil pastel. Since she did not know what to draw, I suggested that she make a picture expressing sadness, adding that sometimes it was helpful to get rid of sad feelings by putting them onto paper.

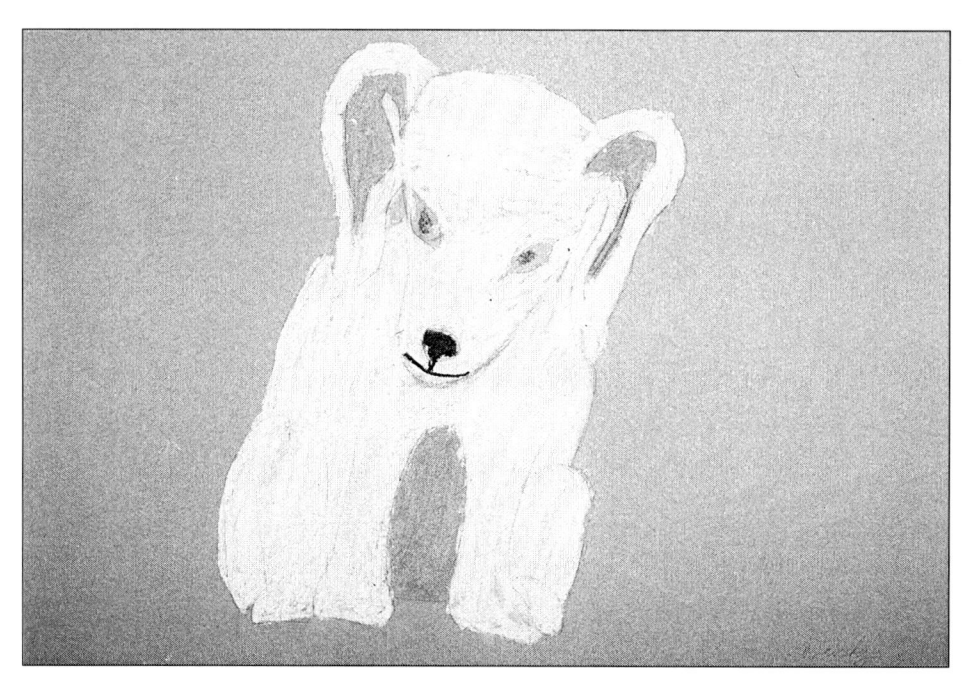

Figure 3.41. *Lucky*, oil pastels by Katja, 12 years.

For a while she seemed to think about it, and then she asked me to draw "Lucky," her white dog (Figure 3.41: "Lucky," oil pastel by Katja, 12 years). "You know, my dog Lucky, when she is sad, she is able to show it so good. Then she would sit in front of you, with a slightly bent head, and look at you with big sad eyes. I miss her so much." Following her description I made the outline drawing. For the rest of the session she worked independently, in silence. When she was blending the colors with her fragile fingers, I had the association of her petting her dog. When she had her final look at the picture, she said: "You were right. I feel much better now. Lucky is so cute. She is such a good friend." It was the only time during the whole program that she used the art-making process in a more conscious way to express feelings.

It took her several weeks to recover. During this time she was working in her usual way with oil pastels, still needing the containment of my outline drawings. The themes remained narrow, with mainly animals (dogs, cats, rabbits), rarely human figures (e.g., a swimming girl). Knowing that animals often unconsciously represent small children, I was wondering if that was her expression of her need for protection.

When she felt strong enough, she declared that she was tired of oil pastels and wanted to learn something new. I listed the options. Finally, I introduced collage with photographic images to her and she looked through my image collection, choosing mainly landscapes and pets. As usual at the beginning of something new, she showed some insecurity, but made her mind up quickly about the theme: one collage about landscapes (Figure 3.42: Untitled, collage by Katja, 12 years), one about pets.

With great pleasure she cut the images and recombined them on a huge piece of paper. By overlapping them she tried to make sure that she didn't leave any gaps. As with Emma, 13 years of age, she seemed to need to keep control over the situation, and to avoid any kind of unpredictabilities. Obviously, as a severely ill teenager, she was fighting with enough unpredictabilities in her life. For the whole session she worked with great concentration, saying little. Her main concern seemed to be to make sure all gaps were closed and to choose matching colors. As usual she did not want to give any associations. "I was just recombining all the landscapes I liked," was her explanation. I wondered if that was her way to extend her own horizon and to go beyond her restricted freedom, at least in fantasy.

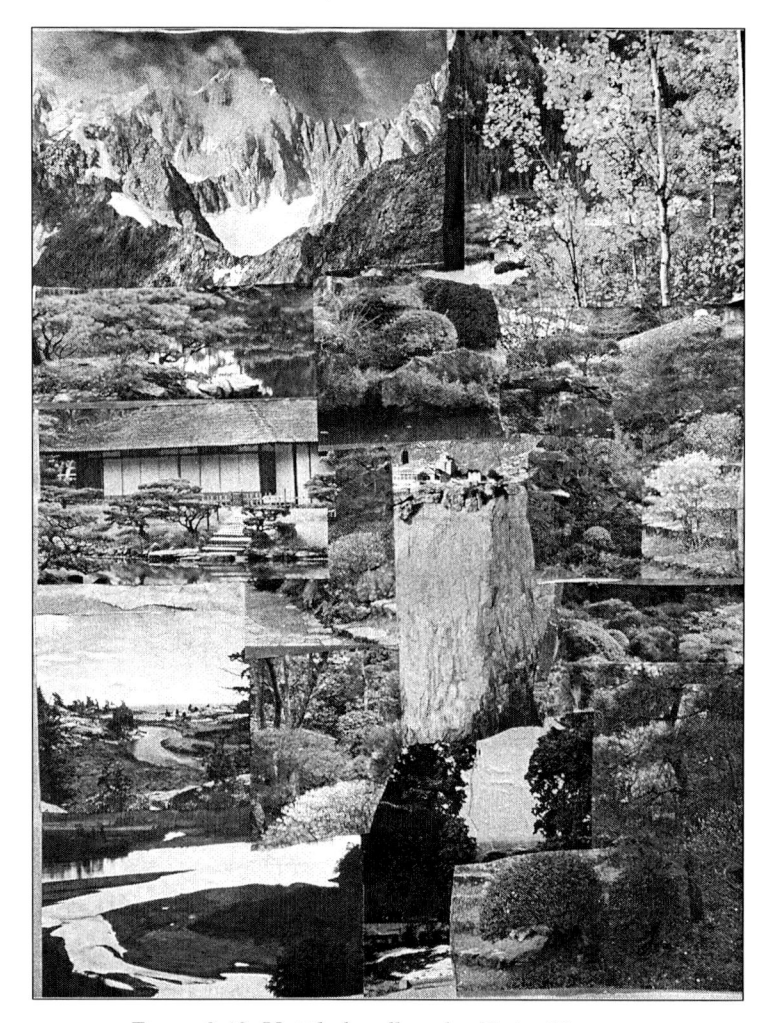

Figure 3.42. Untitled, collage by Katja, 12 years.

During the following few weeks she made another two collages: one about landscapes with water (seashores, river, lakes, glaciers, etc.) and one about dogs. Both were much looser in the sense that she would allow the paper to shine through. During all these weeks it was again striking as to just how much glue she used. All her collages were soaking wet by the time they were finished; and there was glue everywhere on her table, the bed sheet, her body. She was obviously enjoying this process to the fullest extent.

The following session she was waiting for me. She decided to make a watercolor painting of spring flowers (Plate 8. "Spring Flowers," watercolor by Katja, 12 years, p. 48).

She asked me to show her how to do it on a separate piece of paper. Step by step she copied tulips, daisies and roses, in different colors. She was working surprisingly autonomous, without talking a lot. The picture was well balanced. As usual she did not give any association. But with pride she stated that for this piece I did not touch the paper a single time. It was all done by herself. Obviously it was about enhancing her self-confidence.

The following session she wanted to make something really new. I made several suggestions. She immediately went for papier-maché, planning a bowl (Figure 3.43: Bowl, papier-maché by Katja, 12 years).

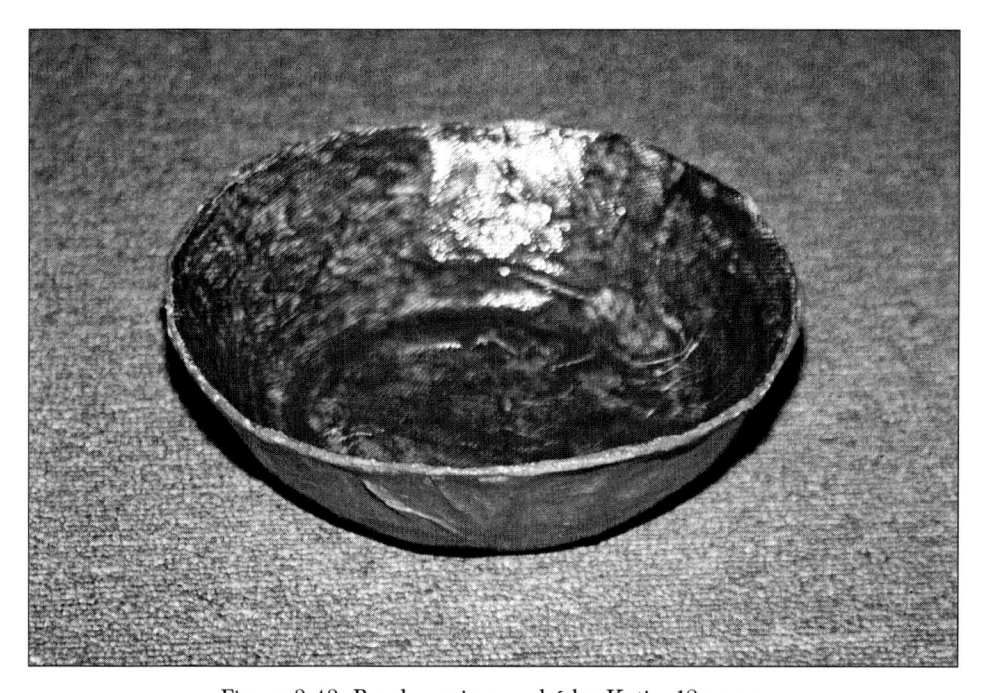

Figure 3.43. Bowl, papier-maché by Katja, 12 years.

Using a basket wrapped in tinfoil as support, I showed her how to do it. She quickly took over. For a while she was doing all the work on her own, as if she wanted to proof her capability. Then she asked me if I could tear the paper strips because it would hasten the process if she could concentrate on gluing. A well-balanced, intense teamwork developed, one in which she used huge amounts of glue and worked in deep concentration. Except for discussing technical points, there was no talking. By the end of the session, she was exhausted.

It took her three sessions to finish her bowl, including the painting of it. During the third of these sessions, but before she started to paint the bowl, I had to start termination (lasting the last six weeks of the program). As with all the other children, I put stickers on a calendar to indicate the countdown. Katja's immediate response to termination was a short period of absolute withdrawal. While she was painting her bowl she did not say a single word and avoided any eye contact. I sensed that it was not the moment to explore her feelings, but rather to let her know about my feelings of sadness, adding that saying goodbye was always difficult for everybody, but that maybe we could help each other. I did not get an answer. She obviously needed time to process her own feelings. I do not know if the colors she used (earthy brown for the inside, sky blue for the outside) represented her feelings, but I had the feeling that her bowl was another metaphor for her need for containment.

Finally when she was done with the painting, she seemed to awake from a bad dream. With sad eyes she made long eye contact with me, somehow letting me know in a non-verbal way that it was not the time to talk about separation. Then she declared that for the rest of the time she wanted to make something really special. My sense was that she wanted to do something that reminded her of the time we shared. We spent time going through the list of available materials. Then with a big smile she told me that she would like to make her own dream catcher (Figure 3.44: "My Personal Dream Catcher," by Katja, 12 years). Was she hoping to keep the bad dream of separation under control with this?

Although we were almost at the end of the session, she wanted to start the dream catcher right away. I had the feeling she needed this extra time. It was as if she had to make sure that I would come back the next time – and the way to ensure that would be to have an unfinished piece of art.

As usual, her initial fear was that she wouldn't be able to do it. So I was surprised by how quickly she learned the knotting and how dexterous her fragile fingers were working.

We started the next session with the termination ritual, which she accomplished like she would do with her homework. She wanted to get right to work decorating her "own and private" dream catcher. Choosing all kinds of materials that we found in Linda's craft cupboard, she carefully planned the decoration. For the whole session she was absorbed in her work and did not talk a lot. When she was done she had a long satisfied look. She was wondering if a dream catcher really worked. I told her that the Natives say that one has to believe in one's own dream catcher to make it work. She seemed to like this answer.

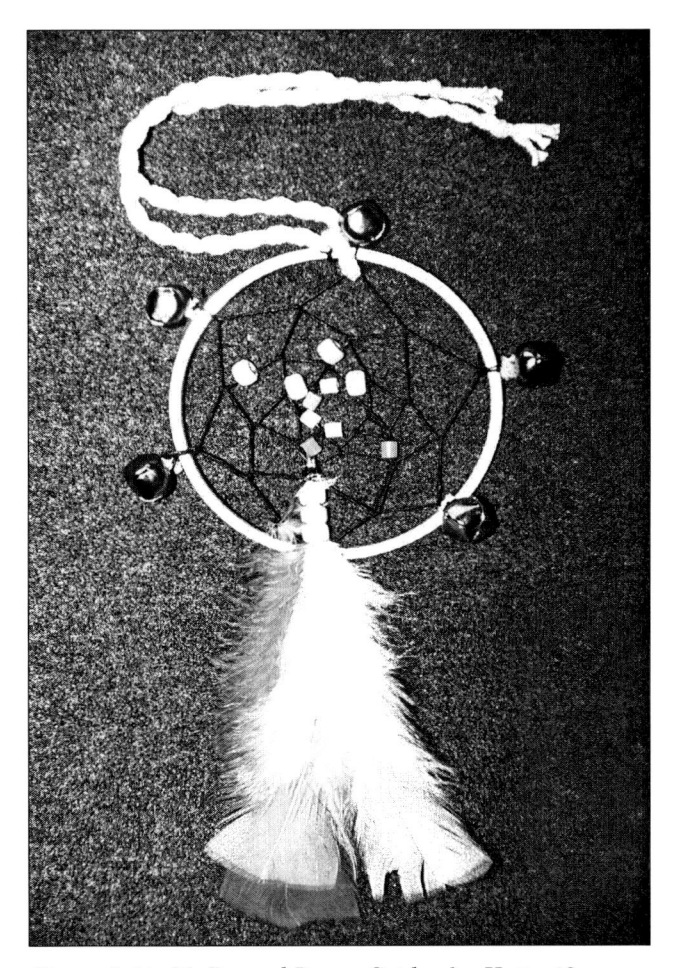

Figure 3.44. *My Personal Dream Catcher*, by Katja, 12 years.

To me her choice and combination of colors was very interesting since they were the same colors all the teenage girls in my program seemed to prefer.

For the last few weeks of the program Katja was the one who reminded me of the termination ritual. I had the feeling it was something she had to accomplish in order to get it out of her mind for the rest of the session. Several times I tried to pick up the termination theme again, but apparently it seemed to be a bigger problem for me than for her.

At each session she had a quick look through her folder to check what kind of art piece it needed to be complete. I wondered if termination for her meant finally being able to take her folder home; and whether she really understood the full extent of termination in the sense that we would not meet anymore. Or did the fact that she cared so much for her folder make it, in a sense, a "transitional object?" I addressed the theme. On the surface she seemed to understand; but I had no idea what it looked like inside her.

In order to complete her folder she added another oil pastel drawing of a girl. This time she did not want me to touch the paper, but just to give her some hints on a separate piece of paper. Suddenly I developed a deep feeling of relief. I understood that she had used these last weeks of termination to wrap up the program by going through these major art techniques, but now was working on her own – her way to prove to herself and to me that now she was capable of working more independently. She definitely had gained self-confidence.

For the second last session she decided to make a pencil drawing (Figure 3.45: "Running Dog with Her Puppy," pencil drawing by Katja, 12 years). She wanted to draw the animals on her own. But in need of help, she asked me to give her some hints using a separate piece of paper. For the first, bigger dog she had to invest her full concentration. There was not a lot of time to talk. After she was done with it, she quickly decided to add a second smaller one – a mom and her puppy. This time she developed some security, which allowed her to talk. She told me about her ten-year-old dog, "Lucky," and how she would like to have another one later because they are the most reliable creatures on earth.

I wondered if the two dogs running back towards the "past" side of the picture were symbolizing the two of us. Somehow the picture was mirroring her wish to go back to the past, when we were still working together. Katja only now allowed her sadness about separation to emerge. At the same time I got a sense of her disappointment about being abandoned because I was not as reliable as a dog would have been. On the other hand, when she was talking about her old dog, she gave a clear message about her capability to enjoy the moment. She obviously was fully aware that each moment (or life) would come to an end at some point. But with her plans to buy a new dog to replace "Lucky" she made it clear that there was always a way that led towards the future.

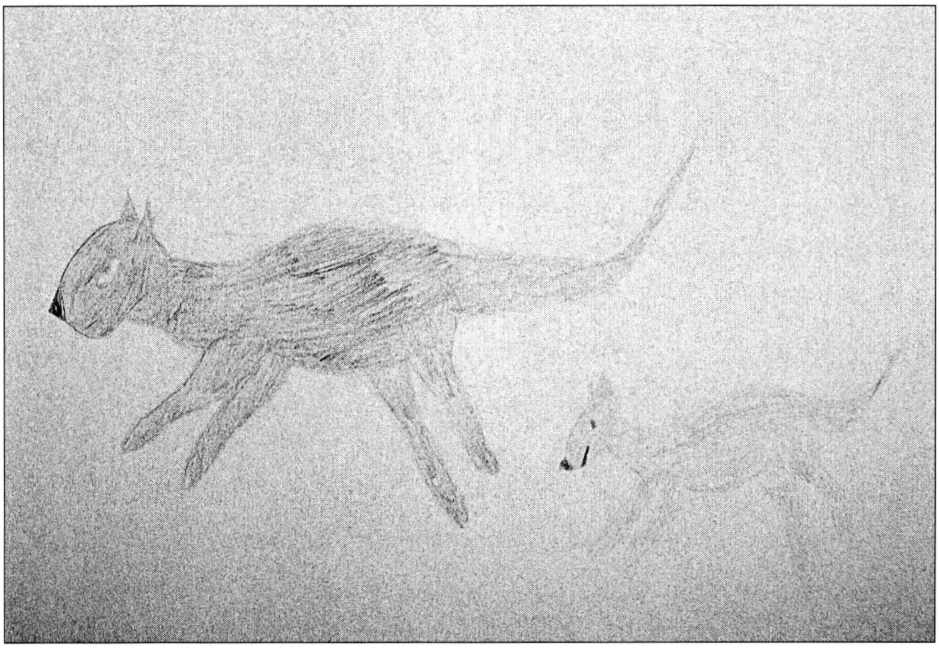

Figure 3.45. *Running Dog with her Puppy*, pencil drawing by Katja, 12 years.

I was surprised by her huge emotional development as compared to the insecure and helpless girl of nine months ago.

For her last session we had to add another hour. She was totally happy with her completed folder, but she absolutely needed to make two more things. I made a comment about how hard it was to let go, and that this extra time was maybe a means to postpone the painful moment of separation. "Maybe, but . . . " was her answer. She told me about her dream catcher: she had to give it to her sister because Julie was having real bad dreams. Now Julie was fine, and Katja was the one having bad dreams. So she desperately needed another dream catcher. This was the goal for the first part of the session. I was surprised how fast and decisive she was working on her own. When she was done, she liked it even better than the first one.

For the second half of the session she had to add another oil pastel drawing to her folder: one she made herself without any help. On a big piece of paper she drew a round glass container with a huge ardent red goldfish. She definitely wanted to show me that now she was able to make it on her own. When I asked her for associations, she listed the general meanings of the goldfish in Chinese culture (long life, etc.). To me this last picture was a metaphor for her amazing emotional growth and maturity. This big goldfish with a smiling face and a marvelous veil-like tail, heading to the right (future) side of the picture, reflected her. On the one hand she was well-contained by the bowl aquarium, but on the other hand this aquarium was definitely now too small for her, and she needed more space. She grew out of her initial secure base, and needed more space in order to move on.

To me it was very important for the two of us to have this extra time in her last session. How could a final piece better express and summarize the progress Katja made over the previous nine months?

SUMMARY

Twelve-year-old Katja was, after initial difficulties, very well able to connect with me. She always was a shy and withdrawn child, suffering of very low self-esteem and self-confidence as a result of her severe physical illness with a lot of complications. Although she loved doing art and crafts, she often would not trust herself to be capable of doing it. She used her art to exercise decision-making and to enhance self-confidence and independence, using me as her auxiliary ego to contain her. In this holding environment of art therapy she was able to develop self-confidence and to gain autonomy. Finally I found her definitely to have gained ego-strength.

7. Nadja, Female, 13 Years

Description of the Client

Nadja was a skinny thirteen-year-old girl of average height. Her straight black hair and brown skin tone were proofs of her Indian-East African origin. She seemed to be still far away from entering puberty, with absolutely no signs of secondary female features. She had a high baby-like voice and tended to talk fast.

Nadja was a bright adolescent with good academic skills, despite interruptions at school due to her illness. She had a healthy curiosity and liked to spend time trying and exploring recipes and guidelines of arts and crafts books and magazines. Her dream was to become a fashion designer or an artist. She liked to share and teach her experiences and discoveries, and to discuss with people she trusted. She was warm and engaging and made quick eye contact. She was capable of good back-and-forth communication.

Her initial shy and child-like behavior of a small girl changed with time to a more demanding-manipulative and at times defiant behavior, and finally in a more interactive behavior between good friends. She had a highly developed creativity and an age-appropriate abstract thinking.

Her mood was even. She had good impulse control, and never really displayed anger. Although she never showed openly her feelings, she was able to express and explore them through art, and therefore, became more aware of them. She did not seem to have a good feeling for her limitations and tended to overwhelm herself with tasks, demanding then for external help and support.

Her positive thinking fueled her explorative behavior, and she had a healthy strength to take risks. She exhibited a narrow range of themes, being mainly interested in underwater creatures, mermaids and other cartoon figures. Very rarely she would follow my suggestions, and totally refused to accomplish one of my directives (tree drawing, bridge drawing). Over the time of our art therapy program she started to use her cartoon figures in a more metaphoric way to express her feelings and explore her issues.

Nadja's strongest defense mechanisms were resistance in passive-aggression and demanding-manipulative behavior, especially when she feared losing control over the situation. She definitively had a tendency to displace and suppress negative, intolerable feelings like anger, aggression, and anxiety. Finally, she would show a childish-helpless or stubborn-defiant behavior when not getting enough attention. Often I had the feeling that her almost compulsive striving for perfection was another defensive behavior to deflect unbearable feelings.

Social History

Nadja was a good student in grade seven. Due to her open and friendly way in encountering people she was well-embedded and popular in her class, despite her frequent absence from school.

Nadja was the younger of two children, and had an eighteen-year-old brother. Both parents were of East African origin (Kenya) with Indian background and Islamic religion, both immigrated as young people. Her father immigrated as an adolescent boy with his family (parents and two brothers). Together they founded the TV/Radio supply store Nadja's father (the youngest of the siblings) would take over later, after the death of his father and the retirement of his brothers. Nadja's mother immigrated on her own in her twenties leaving her family back in Kenya. The two families knew each other in Africa and the marriage was prearranged when they were still children. Mother was always busy as a housewife and mother.

Nadja's brother was an extreme preterm baby with a lot of problems, but later doing excellent. I met him several times visiting his sister. He was involved and interested in his sister's well-being, being well aware of the somehow close and controlling relationship between mother and sister. Apparently he tried several times to open his mother's eye (according to herself).

The family lived in its own condo and seemed to be financially well-stabilized.

Nadja's mother was an engaged, warm maternal woman. With her friendly way of encountering people we made quick contact and were able to build a trustful relationship. She often shared openly her concerns with me and seemed to understand very well what art therapy was about. Usually she waited for me together with Nadja, but then left us alone for the duration of the session. It took me a long time to become aware of the controlling influence she had on Nadja, often narrowing her space of decision-making.

Nadja was always a fragile skinny child suffering of eating problems. As soon as she was started with spoon meals the struggle between mother and daughter around food started, and presently continues. Despite Nadja's 13 years of age mother and daughter still had a very close, almost symbiotic relationship, leaving each other very little space. Nadja had to drop out the summer dialysis camp because of homesickness, mother called several times to make sure that everything was fine with her daughter. Both seemed to need a lot of control over each other, food and eating seemed to be the stage where the power struggle took place.

Nadja did not seem to have a lot of peer contacts outside of her family, beside the interrupted school visits.

Medical History

Nadja was born on term after a normal pregnancy. She was always a healthy child with normal developmental milestones until the age of eleven when her kidney problems started. With her above-average intelligence she was always an excellent student. Even during the last two years she was able to keep up her education, despite her long and frequent school absence.

About two years before we met, her illness started with a heavy diarrhea and nausea, to the point she could not leave the washroom. After ten days she had to be hospitalized because of exhaustion including loss of consciousness. At the hospital they found an end-stage renal failure due to a rheumatologic disease which attacks through its autoantibodies kidneys, brain and lungs. In Nadja's case the lungs were not involved. But she was in coma for about 10 days, and the doctors prepared the parents for a possible death, when she suddenly started to awake from the coma and recover again. Her kidneys were lost and she needed hemodialysis. But her brain (including walking, speech and intellectual skills) recovered totally step-by-step over a period of two months. She spent several months of her rehabilitation time at a pediatric rehabilitation center. During this time she was started on peritoneal dialysis. After one year of peritoneal dialysis she came back to the hospital for hemodialysis. The failure of peritoneal dialysis was due to more and more unbearable abdominal pain during the treatment. Her end-stage renal failure was always well under control due to her exemplary compliance in medication as well as in diet and fluid intake restrictions. She was very aware and careful about all the potentially toxic substances and was almost compulsively wearing gloves to work with art materials.

Towards the end of the art therapy program, Nadja underwent an extended testing in preparation for kidney transplant. Since her family did not want to be tested, she was put on the transplant list for a cadaveric kidney. (Her mother did not want to be tested, knowing that she will always be in charge for Nadja, and therefore, having to be healthy and intact.)

One month later Nadja had to have a gastric tube implanted, because she had lost too much weight and her calorie intake was still too low, especially in context with her stressful chronic physical illness, and a pending kidney transplantation.

Art Therapy Process and Artwork

The art therapy program lasted for 48 sessions. I started to work with her as soon as the hemodialysis was installed. Although she was happy to discontinue peritoneal dialysis, it took her some time to adjust to the different schedule of the hemodialysis routine. According to the social worker's request, in agreement with my supervisor, I started to work with Nadja twice a week. Included in the introduction of the art therapy program we fixed with Nadja and her mother, to switch back to once a week as soon as possible or the latest for the last ten weeks of the program's termination phase.

By reviewing Nadja's art I realized that we went through four main stages over the period of nine months. In each stage she seemed to express and explore a particular main issue, related to a particular transference and inducing a particular countertransference.

The *first stage* of forming a trustful working alliance lasted for about six weeks.

After the introduction and demonstration of the available art material Nadja decided to start with her first piece (Figure 3.46: Untitled, mixed media collage by Nadja, 13 years).

For the whole session she was working with all kinds of art supplies, combining everything, trying and changing ideas, but always using pencil and eraser first to keep control over her piece of art. To my surprise twenty minutes after we met each other, she engaged me into her process of art-making by giving me small controllable tasks to fulfill. Finally she got her cartoon of Mr. Happy Potato Head jumping a rope under a rainbow, at the shore of a lake with fishes. The picture was drawn onto white paper and in a second session glued into a rainbow frame onto an orange paper. Everything was very colorful and nicely done. Even the rainbow had the exact number and follow-up of colors, as she was taught at school.

For the whole session she was working very concentrated and controlled, but appeared to be in a hurry because she wanted to finish that piece. I had a hard time terminating the first session, and that would remain so for the rest of the program. I immediately sensed her need for attention, and her attempt to be perfect and pleasant. Her first picture was a very colorful and nicely done piece, an interesting combination of spontaneity and rational planning, following the rules of aesthetics – hiding a lot of unconscious things.

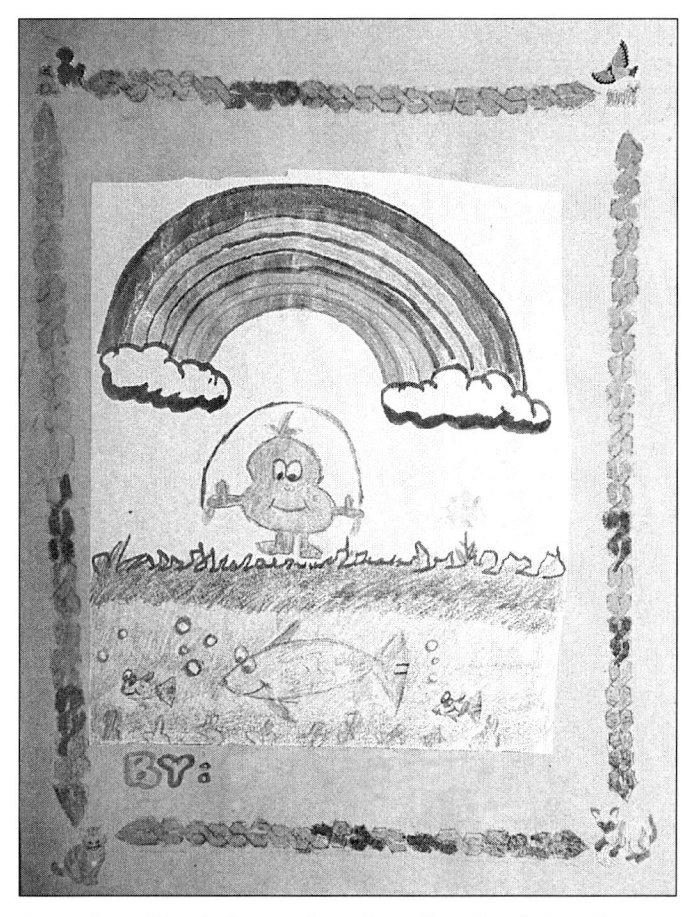

Figure 3.46. Untitled, mixed media collage by Nadja, 13 years.

The following session she wanted to finish the rainbow frame for her first piece. Eventually she finished the frame by adding some stickers. While she was adding stickers to the corner of the frame, she told me about her sticker collection. I had the feeling that by adding these stickers she was trying to close the fence even tighter, in order not to let escape anything or to let people come too close – her attempt to keep control over the situation, her need for protection. Although at the surface she showed a very spontaneous and direct way of working, I could sense her unconscious insecurity and anxiety. Then for the rest of the session she began with another Mr. Happy Potato Head onto white paper, starting with a pencil drawing and coloring it with watercolors. She spent the rest of the session mixing a skin color with paint, asking me for help with this difficult task. She seemed to be very ambitious and hard to satisfy. Her plan was to cut Mr. HPH out and to use it for another collage, which she never did.

As I learned, Mr. Happy Potato Head was an ongoing theme, coming up in the most different completions. It took me a while to realize that her preference for cartoons was less a way to displace issues, but more the stage where she would explore them.

The following session Nadja decided to work in clay, an unknown material, which she would use only once for the entire art therapy program (Figure 3.47: "My Mug," clay mug by Nadja, 13 years).

For a long time she was exploring, kneading, flattening and re-kneading again. Several times she tried to make a vase or a plate, but threw it together again. She seemed hard to be satisfied, and obviously had very high expectations. Finally, she managed to make some sort of mug with very thick walls. Again I had a hard time to terminate this session. Telling me that next time the clay will be hard, she tried to extend the session. But I assured her that I would keep the clay mug wet and soft for her until the next session.

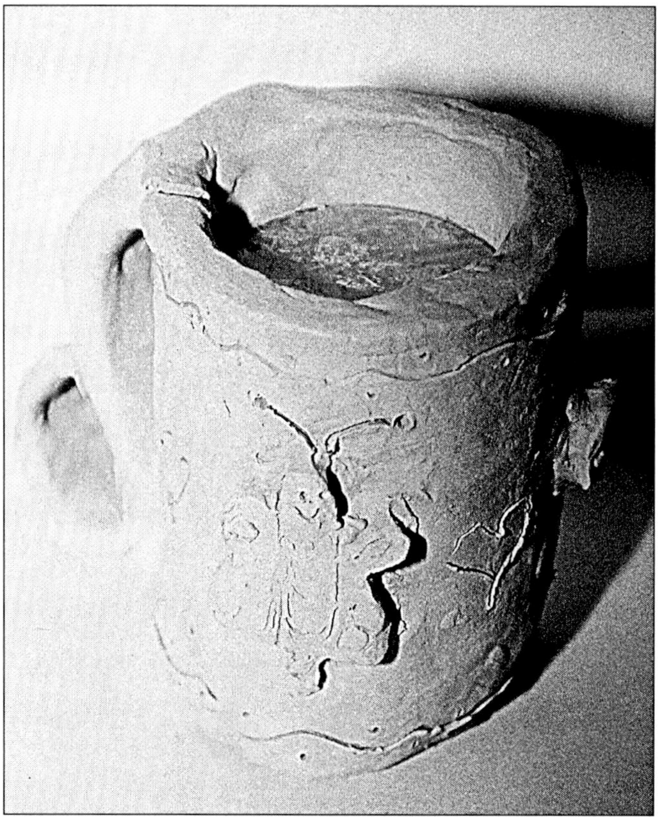

Figure 3.47. *My Mug*, clay mug by Nadja, 13 years.

During this whole session she told me about cooking and baking, about different kitchen tools, and finally about eating and food. At that time I didn't know about the ongoing theme of nutrition and eating problems. It took her two sessions to eventually finish her mug. The second session she added a strong handle, then it was time to make the decoration. She asked me to flatten a piece of clay for her, and started to cut out two butterflies and a sun, which she stuck onto the mug. Then she started to decorate the whole thing by scratching with a toothpick. While she was working she told me about another mug with two seahorses she made at school, but she never fired. She wanted to know if we would fire this piece, but I had to disappoint her in her attempt to make something permanent. She took that information without any problems.

In general I was surprised how easy she was able to overcome disappointments or failures of things she was trying. She never became angry or give up, but would rather look for another solution.

The following session Nadja wanted to work with oil pastels on a huge white piece of paper (Figure 3.48: Untitled, oil pastels by Nadja, 13 years). First she drew a goldfish surrounded with deep blue water, the whole picture the size of a postcard. Then she started to draw Mr. Happy Potato Head in another corner of the same big white paper. She told me that she wanted to recycle the whole piece of paper and she started to cover the rest of the page with red-blue-purple abstract shapes. Then she covered these shapes with a thick layer of black oil pastel. Finally, she started to scratch into the black surface and to reveal Mr. Happy Potato Head, another fish and a sun. Then she started to cut these three elements of images into smaller individual pieces, adding fancy borders. She declared she might use them later for a collage, which she never did. Several times during the program she would repeat this strange working process of starting with scattered, thematically independent drawings on a big piece of paper, to eventually fragment the whole piece. I was wondering about the significance of this behavior, but never found a satisfying answer.

This was the session when she started to wear surgical gloves for whatever technique she was working with. She told me that she wanted to protect herself from dangerous substances, an obsessive behavior she would keep for the rest of the program.

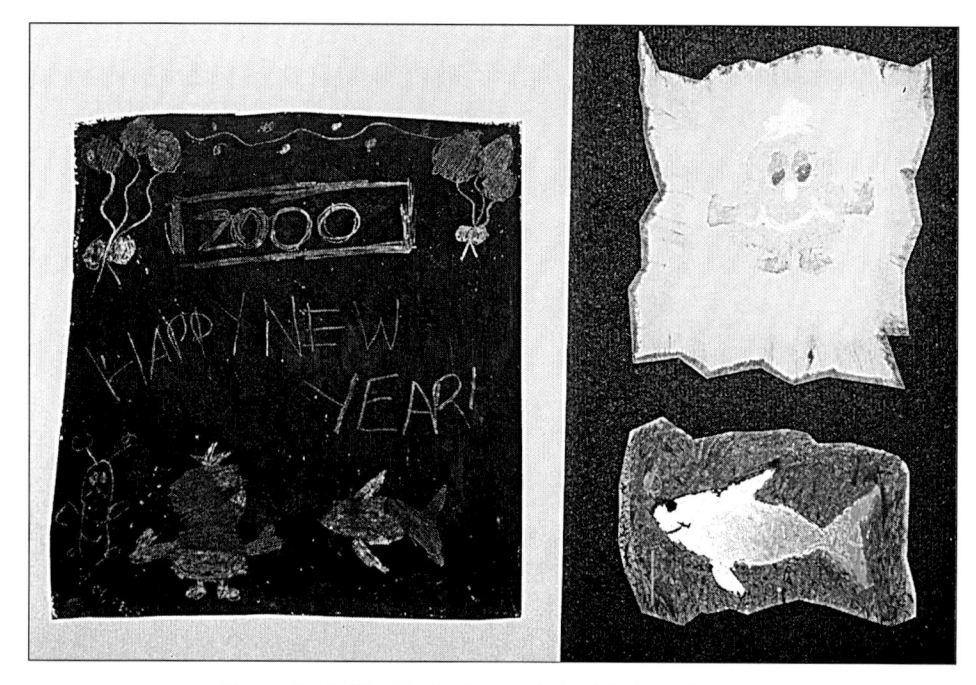

Figure 3.48. Untitled, oil pastels by Nadja, 13 years.

While she was drawing she told me about the pending surgery the same afternoon, when she had to have the tube removed in her abdomen that she still had from her peritoneal dialysis time. Openly she told me how scared she was due to the bad experiences she had last time. At the same time she was drawing all these happy and funny creatures. There was a big discrepancy between the content of her verbal and her visual communication.

I asked her for her association for fishes. But she did not have any, she did not like fishes as animals, nor as pets because they are boring. Nevertheless, it started to be an ongoing theme, maybe as main participants in her underwater scenery that she was so interested in, and she would use in a metaphorical way later.

The following session Nadja wanted to try chalk pastels (Figure 3.49: "Molly and Paul Holding Hands," chalk pastels by Nadja, 13 years). I was surprised when she started to draw and color with pastels directly, without using the safety of pencil and eraser. Never before I did see her draw in such a spontaneous way.

After having divided the piece of paper in half with a purple vertical line, she continued her drawing by adding all kinds of fruits. I asked her for her associations of the fruits, but she could not give me any. She added that in general she was a terrible eater, and that she was eating very little and very selective like a small child.

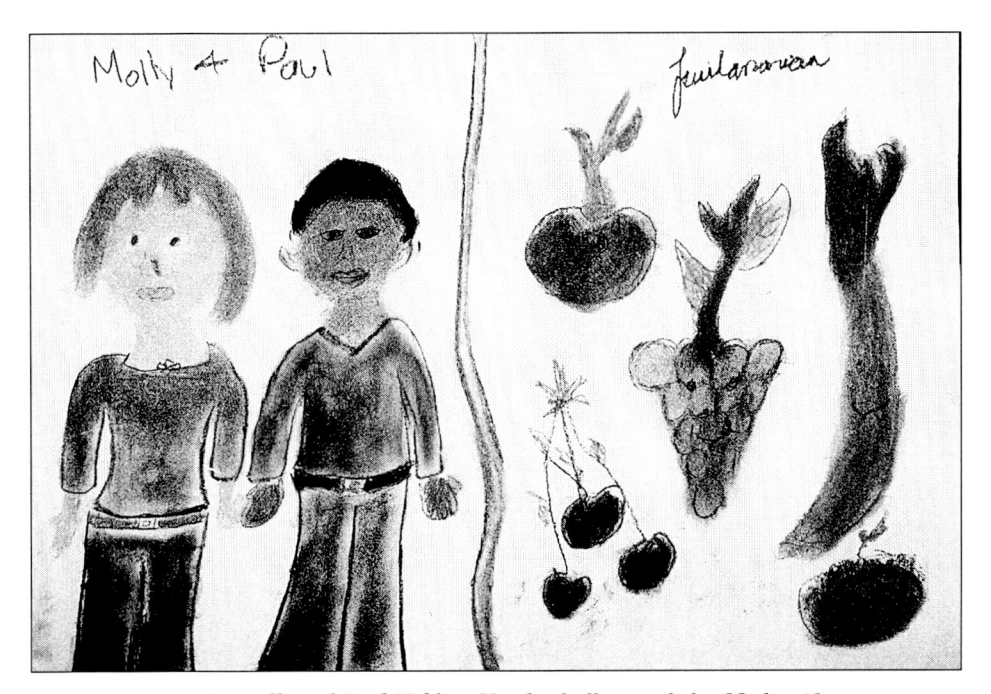

Figure 3.49. *Molly and Paul Holding Hands*, chalk pastels by Nadja, 13 years.

While she was drawing these pictures she told me spontaneously the whole story of her disease starting at the age of 11, and how she recovered completely except for the kidneys, and after having been given up for lost. The one and a half years of peritoneal dialysis were a terrible time because she suffered a lot of pain. That was why they switched her to hemodialysis.

For the first time she was loose enough to give up the control of pencil and eraser, and for the first time she drew human figures and not cartoons. I could sense a lot of duality in this picture – the two independent pictures on either side of the page and the two human figures of different races.

The following session Nadja wanted to work with "real paint," and how I learned later she meant "aquarelles" by that (Figure 3.50: Untitled, watercolor by Nadja, 13 years). Again she did not use pencil and eraser to control the process, but went into her painting with the pencil later to set some accents. During the whole process of painting she made me mix her colors, since we had only primary and secondary colors. After a while I made a comment about her keeping me busy, just to make her aware about the demanding behavior she was showing. Her tough answer was: "Isn't that what it is about here?" I was too surprised about this sudden arise of defiance to give an answer. Then I asked her if this female captain was her. Again her defiant answer was "No! Do I have blonde hair?" So I realized, it is not the time to ask questions. I was wondering about this fair female captain who apparently just left an island, leading her sailing boat towards the right (future) side of the picture. Was this her metaphor for leaving the secure base in order to head towards a new future, hoping to discover and explore new realms?

Then she turned the paper around, switched to chalk pastels and started a new small drawing about a girl and a small boy. Her spontaneous explanation was: "That's a girl teasing this boy. He is not her brother, nor her boyfriend. She is just teasing him because he is so small." Again she turned the page around and drew another small scene of two girls holding hands. "These are two good friends. They are mad because the boyfriend of one girl left her for another girl. And now they are talking together and making plans of revenge." Nadja was not in the mood to add more; that was it. Again her final piece included several thematically independent scenes on one piece of paper. This time she did not cut them, but separated them by changing the orientation of the drawings. I was wondering if this was the reflection of the tension she was obviously experiencing.

In this session she reached the top of her demanding behavior and I felt I had to make a comment about it. Her reaction was to get back with even more defiance and passive aggression. For the first time I could sense her real self with its issues. I was wondering about her changing the direction of her drawings, and the stories she told me in that context. Did she sense there was a changing in direction within the art therapy program as well? It definitively was her way to express anger and aggression.

During this first stage of building a trustful working alliance we were able to know each other and to become attuned to each other. Nadja discovered different kinds of art material until she found her favorite technique she felt comfortable with. During this period she did not only explore different supplies, but was testing boundaries as well – sometimes in an appropriate way, sometimes with an undertone of demand and manipulation.

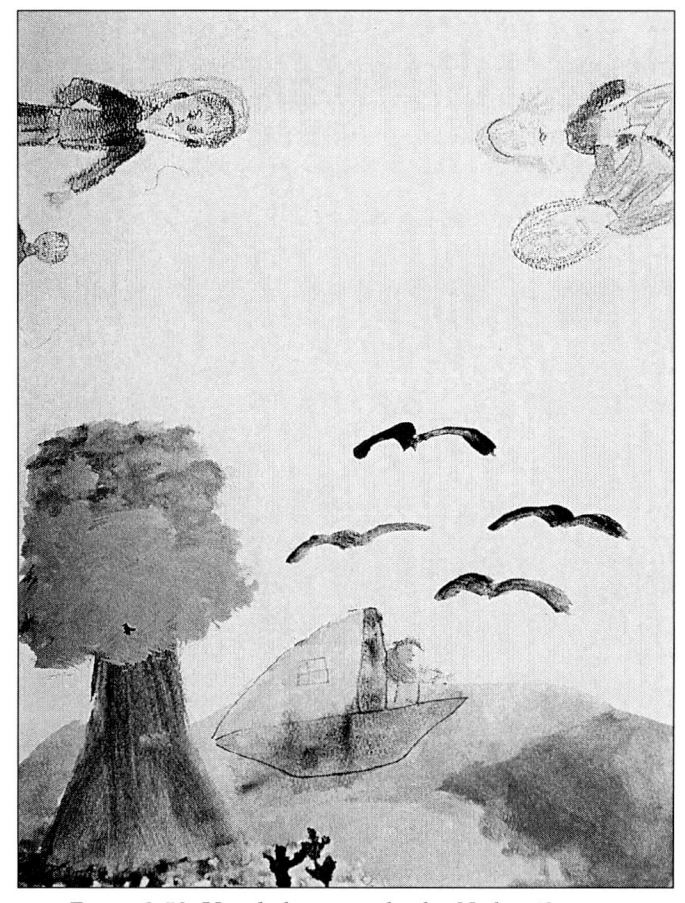

Figure 3.50. Untitled, watercolor by Nadja, 13 years.

The *second stage* of exploring adolescent issues lasted about six weeks. One of the following sessions Nadja decided to use chalk pastels (Figure 5.51: "Styles of Ways of Clothing, Styles of Hair," chalk pastels by Nadja, 13 years). She divided a white piece of paper in half by drawing a vertical line. On the left-hand side she drew "Styles of ways of clothing," on the top right-hand side "Styles of hair." For the whole time she was working very concentrated and very carefully, without talking a lot. Very briefly she mentioned that she would like to become a fashion designer and to create her own collection.

That day she was withdrawn and somehow thoughtful, with an underlying hint of sadness. She did not want to share any of her sorrows, but included me into her art-making process by asking me for help in blending colors. Despite her depressed mood she was able to have a very engaged and engaging teamwork.

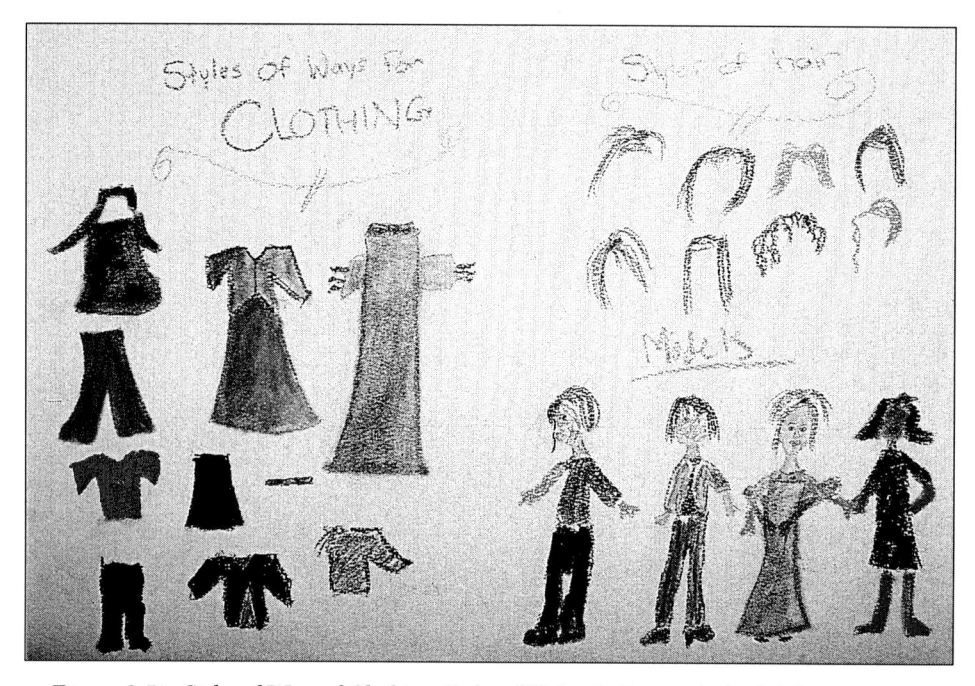

Figure 3.51. *Styles of Ways of Clothing, Styles of Hair*, chalk pastels by Nadja, 13 years.

It took her two sessions to finish this piece. The next session she was again fine and in a good mood, almost high-spirited. While she was finishing her previous picture by adding four models wearing her own collection of clothes she created last time, she was talking all the time touching several themes: Comparing her parents driving styles, describing the area of the city they are living, the school she went to on and off, and so forth. When I asked her if she had friends, she shrugged her shoulder and told me about her brother's friends instead. I sensed her social isolation. After a while of silence she told me about a good friend of hers who came from Bangladesh, but who was not allowed to immigrate and had to go back. "All my good friends have to leave again," she said with a meaningful and sad face.

For the rest of the session we talked about her models wearing her own fashion collection, and how she would like to cloth herself – she likes to cover her neck in a decent way, whereas her mother would allow her more feminine "risky" clothes. I was wondering about power-control struggle between the two of them. Or was that her expression of her feelings around the development of body image and sexuality, a metaphor for her conflicts about her developing body shape and sexuality?

Case Histories and Artwork 161

Although she was fine the following session, she did not talk a lot during this session. After she ordered the material she wanted to use (chalk pastels, pencil crayons and scissors) she started to work quietly and very concentrated (Figure 3.52: "Under Sea," chalk pastels, by Nadja, 13 years).

After having written the title "Under Sea" she started to draw a nice little mermaid with red hair, Ariel as I learned later. Then she added several sea creatures like seahorse, starfish, fish, squid and a shell with a pearl. Finally she added a shipwreck, making me guess about its name. She asked me if I had watched the movie *Titanic* and how I liked it, mentioning that she did not really like it. To finish the piece she added a jumping dolphin under a laughing sun on the right half of the paper.

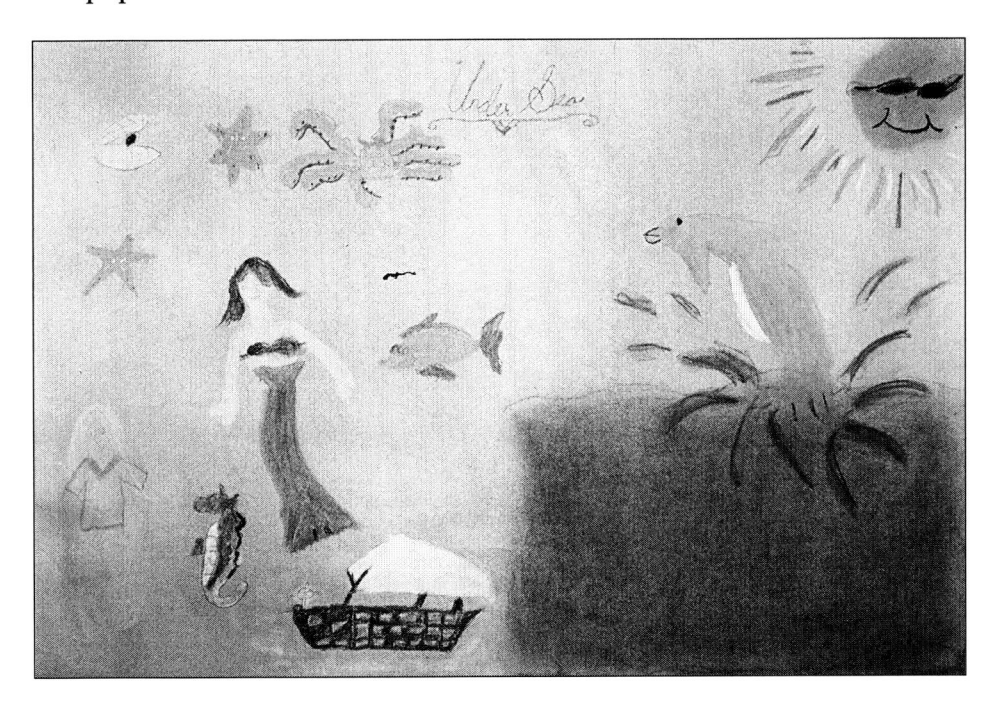

Figure 3.52. *Under the Sea*, chalk pastels by Nadja, 13 years.

All the underwater items did not really interact with each other. I did not get the sense of a story. The whole drawing was nicely done, but somehow lifeless and static. Only with the jumping dolphin was there life in the picture. She did not give me any association. Again I was wondering about this duality: static versus dynamic, below versus above water level, reality versus dream world. Was that her way to extend her restricted world in order to explore her feelings and issues?

The following session, the unit was very busy and loud. Nevertheless Nadja seemed to be able to concentrate.

She asked for a white paper and chalk pastels and started right away to draw single independent scenes the size of a postcard, all around the paper (Plate 9: Untitled, chalk pastels by Nadja, 13 years, p. 49), a red goldfish in dark blue water, a colorful butterfly and three schematic birds, a green caterpillar named "Squimmy," a cute little dog sitting on top of the earth. All these small scenes did not have any connection with each other. Nadja was even stressing that fact by turning the paper over and over again, and giving different drawing directions. After a while she asked me if I was bored. I definitively denied, but admitted that I was confused by all these different drawings, turning the paper, and being distracted by all the noise around us. Somehow I had the feeling she could not concentrate as well, but would not admit it.

Suddenly the full energy went back into her and with energetic strokes she started to draw a green alien standing on top of a yellow-ochre globe. Surrounding this scene she drew two mermaids, one nice and happy looking, the other with a very angry appearance, and finally a "merman" with a rose and a parcel in his hands. Whereas I was an inactive observer for the first part of the session, for the second part she engaged me again in helping her with blending colors. When she finished the picture she made me take a blank sheet of paper and write down her story.

"The Mermaid Story"

"Olivia met a boy named Mark and they were best friends. But one day another girl Angela interfered with their relationship. Olivia and Mark separated for a while. Then Angela and Mark hung out always together. And Olivia was kind of jealous. But she left it alone. Mark realized Angela was not a good friend. So Mark thought Olivia was a good friend and wanted to get back together again.

To be continued. . . ."

By Nadja (adding her own signature).

In addition to the exploration of body image and sexuality as part of Nadja's identity, the often strongly connected feelings of jealousy and rivalry were obviously coming up. With her story about the mermaids she created a metaphor for her own conflicts.

After having a longer look at her piece, she decided to cut it and make all the small scenes for little postcards in a future collage, leaving only the mermaid scene intact. She told me that in future she wanted to continue with this story, maybe even to write a book.

I was wondering about her tendency to fragment her picture, stressing it even by cutting them. Was that a sign for her confusion that I was picking up as a projective identification? Was she exploring different elements of herself in search for her own cohesive identity? Or was she simply trying to develop more freedom, more flexibility by breaking the conventional frame and adding additional dimensions? With this she signalizes her search for independence. A logical next step would be to add a third dimension, like a 3-D work, which would add a tactile component as well.

The next session she was perfectly fine and was waiting for me to continue her mermaid story. She chose her favorite technique and started right away on a white piece of paper (Plate 10: "Family Portrait," chalk pastels by Nadja, 13 years, p. 49).

While she was drawing the family portrait of the two mermaids Olivia (to the right) and Angela (to the left) including their mothers, she told me their story in details. "Olivia and Angela were two good friends since early childhood. Their families knew each other well. Angela's mother is dark, but her father who died centuries ago, was white. That's why she is half-and-half, and she was teased a lot and suffered because of that. But Olivia always took her part. Olivia was teased because of her long arms. So the two girl mermaids stuck together. Angela's mother is very fashion oriented: she colors her hair and applies facial masks, and so on, whereas Olivia's mother is a very humble and nice woman."

I was again wondering about this duality. Reviewing her previous work I am pretty sure that both mermaids including their mothers are part of Nadja. The story of these two so different characters being united in a good friendship, but occasionally struggling with jealousy and competition which is the stage where Nadja was exploring her unconscious issues in search for her own identity, including body image and sexuality. The mothers of the mermaids are just simply exaggerations of their daughters, to make this scenario even more intense.

When Nadja was done with this first picture, she started immediately a second one, continuing the story by adding Mark, the male part to the scenario (Plate 11: "Mark's Story," chalk pastels by Nadja, 13 years, p. 50).

First she drew Mark's sister who was a witch, then Mark as a small "merman" to her feet. Again she told me his story: "Mark got terribly sick and would have died on earth. In order to keep him alive his sister had to transform him into a merman and send him under sea. Both were terribly sad and cried a lot while saying good-bye forever. That is how Mark came into the water." Turning the paper she added Angela's mother with a green facial mask to make a good impression on Mark. In another corner there was their "merdog."

During this session she did not ask me to help her, but included me into her process by telling me the story. By diving into the underwater world Nadja explored her unconscious issues and needs as an adolescent: body image/beauty/femininity, sexuality/ gender role, independence, and finally, search for her identity.

Next session she wanted to immediately continue with her mermaid story, using her beloved chalk pastels. On a white piece of paper she started to draw two worlds – one is our world (left side) and one is the mermaids' world (right side) (Plate 12: "Our World, the Mermaids' World," chalk pastels by Nadja, 13 years, p. 50).

While she was drawing our world she continued telling me the story: There is a beach with human children playing on it. In the shallow water there is the mermaid Angela who is observing the human beings. "You know, for mermaids it is not allowed to go to the beach and look at humans. If the humans see the mermaids these will lose their identity, because human beings tend to sell everything for attraction. And if they fall in love it is even worse because their kids will be half-and-half. Nevertheless, Angela went there, because she is just curious, and likes to take risks."

Then Nadja started to draw the mermaids' world with a huge castle, and Olivia and Mark waiting in front of it. "Olivia and Mark are waiting for Angela. They fixed to meet to play with each other. But Angela did not show up. You know now why. But the two of them are just very disappointed and somehow mad at Angela – and did not know what to do." For a while Nadja continued to describe the mermaids' world with all its richness and peace.

In that session Nadja was defining even clearer the differences in character between the two mermaids: Angela, the curious "bad girl," disobedient, independent and risk-taking girl; Olivia, the calm "good girl," reasonable, but somehow a dependent and boring girl. Listening objectively to Nadja's storytelling, I had the feeling she was more sympathetic with Angela. Definitively the two girls represented two parts of Nadja. The two worlds seemed to be again the stage where Nadja was exploring her needs as an adolescent.

During the *third stage* lasting for about ten weeks, Nadja was exploring the realm of food and eating habits.

The next session she had a very high blood pressure and was not allowed to eat anything salty. Although she did not have symptoms, she was in a bad mood, and I could feel her anger. First she made me prepare chalk pastels and paper, but then she changed her mind and asked for yarn, scissors and cardboard. She wanted to make a snake out of yarn pong-pongs. I immediately learned that I had to revise my definition for art today and remain flexible for whatever she wanted to make. Usually Nadja was making this kind of craft with the child-life specialist. But obviously that day she had chosen to make it with me in art therapy.

For the whole process of making different sizes of cardboard squares, bind them in yarn, cut the yarn into pong-pong and lining them up in a row, she did not talk at all. She was withdrawn in a passive-aggressive behavior and avoided any contact with me. As I expected she did not finish the snake by the end of the session, but wanted to keep it with her, because she wanted to continue it with the child-life specialist. I did not understand what this was all about, but I let her go with that. I never saw the snake again.

What was this strange session all about? Was she just trying to explore some new dimension by entering the more tactile 3-D world? Usually she made clear distinctions between the crafts she made with the child-life specialist and the art she made in art therapy. But today she seemed to try to connect the two of us, as her two important female roles. Maybe we did not only have an important female, but also a peer role in her exploration of her identity, as well. These additional female contacts might help her gaining more independence from her mother, too.

The following session Nadja suffered of flu symptoms and was very tired. When we met she asked me to bring the computer so she could consult the craft channel on the Internet. I told her that I was very bad in computers and that this was more the child-life's domain. She explained to me that she was tired of continuing the mermaid story and wanted to make something three-dimensional with papier-maché. I told her that she would have my full support even without a computer. So together we started to make plans for her next project – a container made of papier-maché with old newspapers, using a balloon as support. Later she wanted to cut it and to have kind of a bowl and a lid, in order to get a container to store candies and to offer them to visitors.

That day she was physically not strong enough to start with the actual piece, but together we made a list with the material she would need next time. That was the beginning of a longer project.

Over the period of the next ten weeks she was working very consistently and patiently at her papier-maché container, showing a lot of ambition and concentration. It took her three weeks to be sure that the surface was strong enough to pop the balloon and to cut the ball in a bottom and a lid. And even then she continued to add more and more layers of newspaper and white tissue paper on the outside and the inside of the two parts of the container. Her main issues seemed to need a strong enough container for all the candies she wanted to put in. The walls ended up to be about half a centimeter in diameter (Figure 3.53: "Mr. Happy Potato Head," papier-maché container by Nadja, 13 years).

During this long week she enjoyed a totally different way of working than the weeks before – she liked to use a lot of glue and make a big mess on her table. For her own sake, as usual, she was wearing surgical rubber gloves all the time. Her way of working had something strange regressive, like a small child who has to make up the stage of being allowed to make a big mess and to take over the control for the extent of the mess. Again, her way to include me into her working process changed from the more observational position of last stage into a more active one as her assistant. It was not her commanding-manipulative attitude of stage one, but an appropriate integration of my person as an extended arm for the things she could not achieve herself because of her restrictions in working space. This stage was characterized by a well-balanced teamwork, leaving a lot of space for verbal sharing.

Her first plan was to make a planet of this round shape, and to fill it with candies. I had the feeling that with the theme of the planet she tried to expand her so restricted own world (restriction in fluid intake, in diet, in bodily activities, in going for holidays, etc.). Later she changed her mind and decided to make Mr. Happy Potato Head with a big mouth, offering the candies out of his mouth to whom may deserve it. Interesting enough she changed her plans for her bowl after the decision for the G-tube implantation, as if she was looking for another way to keep food as a control means, after having lost the control over her own nutrition.

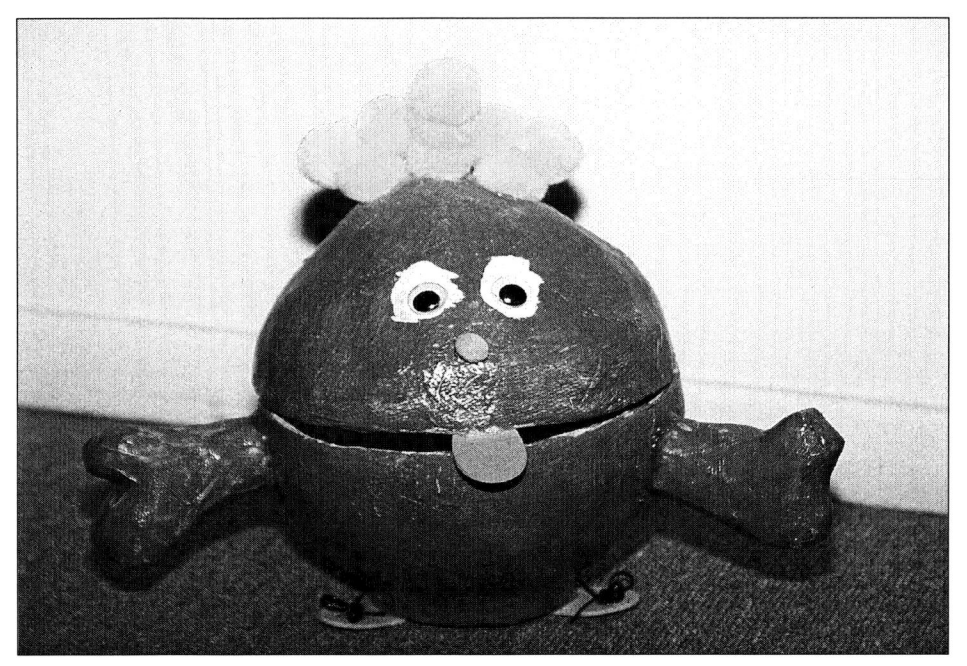

Figure 3.53. *Mr. Happy Potato Head*, papier-maché container by Nadja, 13 years.

During the stage of painting Mr. Happy Potato Head's surface, she spent three sessions just with mixing skin colors, applying it and repainting it anew. For this short period she regressed into her demanding-manipulative behavior again. I was wondering about the importance of this special color. Was it part of her search for her own identity? She obviously needed to feel "right" in her own skin, within her own body, within her own world. It was about the emotional fit, the attachment to herself – another thing she had to discover.

She obviously was enjoying the fact that she was pacing this kind of monotonous work, and she used this time to touch a lot of different themes and issues verbally:

1. *Food, eating, cooking and baking, and her interest in recipes:* An ongoing theme for several sessions was her description how much she liked cooking and baking and exploring new recipes, and her love for cookies! At the same time she taught me a lot about the restriction in diet and fluid intake due to her kidney disease. She was very aware of the treatment concept and was very compliant in following them. She obviously was enjoying the fact that her mother was always looking for new recipes to try new things compatible with the diet, and tasting good enough for her daughter. I sensed that this was the unconscious way Nadja was keeping control over her mother, the typical behavioral pattern in families with anorexic patients.

2. *The time she was working at her candy container was the time the implantation of a G-tube was arranged.* Over the last few months her weight reached a dangerous low level, and she did not eat enough in order to keep it stable. That was why the doctors decided to implant a tube through the skin directly into her stomach, in order to infuse her special high-caloric formula during the night. Each time when we talked about that I could sense her ambivalence between being proud to be a hero and being anxious about the symptoms. Food was the last control she had in her hands, and now she was going to lose this as well. After the implantation, she had difficulties tolerating the formula, and vomitted frequently during the rest of our time together. I was wondering (and trying to mention it with the medical team as well) if this was the ideal treatment, considering the diagnosis of Anorexia nervosa. (Nobody with the exception of me seemed to consider this diagnosis.)

3. *Her few friends:* Only once she told me about her two girlfriends who she met at the dialysis summer camp last year, and with whom she still was in contact. One of them was much older, and her hemodialysis done at another hospital. Nevertheless, they all had a good time and went out together every once in a while.

4. *Her birthday:* For several sessions earlier she told me about all the plans for her birthday party. The session after the party she did not want to talk at all. Obviously it did not turn out the way she expected, but I did not receive further information. Some weeks later in a more enthusiastic way, she told about her brother's birthday, where obviously she acquired more attention than during her own.

5. *The male role in her family:* Nadja released her anger about the laziness of her father, who after work would come home and put his feet

up and let the mother serve him, and now her brother was following this example. At the same time she stressed how much she would help her mother now. Was it jealousy because she had to share her mother's attention with the rest of the family? Was it to elaborate how mature she grew meanwhile? Was it the release of anger about males in her life in relation with her physical illness in general?

6. *Going back to school*: During the long months of unsuccessful peritoneal dialysis, she was not able to go to school because she was too much in pain. But now on hemodialysis she was stable enough to attend school at the dialysis-free days, and that was a big event for her. I sensed her ambivalence between having to give up her spare time and fitting into a school schedule during these days, but having more opportunities to meet peers and to make friends. I think it is a very important step for her even in terms of gaining more independence from her mother.

7. *Starting the test for transplantation*: Her mother did not want her family to be tested as donors with the argument that Nadja would need them intact until the end of her life to support her. I was wondering if that was not another unconscious means of keeping control over her daughter. The longer I was working with Nadja the longer I realized the controlling influence of her mother. Obviously, the controlling behavioral pattern was mutual, which is typical for anorexic patients.

8. *Attending this year's dialysis summer camp*: Nadja told me her bad experiences about her first dialysis camp last year, where her mother had to pick her up because she was so homesick. (Her mother's version was that she had to pick her up because the nurses were not following Nadja's medication properly!) So for this year Nadja had a lot of concerns to try again. For several sessions we talked about that, and how much she changed and matured meanwhile. Finally she decided to give it another trial. Later I learned that this year's camp was an absolute success. "I didn't even have time to be homesick!" was her comment.

During this stage we were asked twice if a nurse student was allowed to observe an art therapy session. Nadja seemed to be enthusiastic about this idea, and quickly took over the role of a "tourist" guide through the session. She explained to the full extent the meaning of art therapy and the difference between craft (where she had to follow given patterns and work exact) and art (where she was allowed to make a mess if she felt, and she was allowed to try things out and to develop her own ideas). She obviously was enjoying the role of a guide or teacher because that would give her the full control over the session. It also provided her an opportunity to show confidence in what she had experienced and learned during art therapy.

As I promised, I took my therapeutic puppet I made in a weekend-workshop for art therapists with me. It was a very strange encounter. Nadja showed a very shy and withdrawn behavior as if she would meet a stranger, but not leaving him out of her eyes. I could sense her ambivalence between being very attracted to him, but at the same time not really knowing if she could trust him. After I put it away and we were working for a whole session, she asked me if it would be possible for her to make her own puppet as well. I encouraged her to think about it and offered her my help. The next time she announced that she wanted to make her own mermaid puppet as soon as Mr. Happy Potato Head was done.

The *fourth and last stage* lasted for about ten weeks. During this time Nadja seemed to explore mainly her body image. She seemed to have very clear ideas about feminine beauty and attraction, which she gave expression by stressing features like very long eyelashes, big blue eyes, full red lips, elegant hands with slim fingers, a small top allowing the belly button to be seen, and so on. It was interesting to see how she was exploring today's teenage fashion directions.

Included in this stage was the phase of termination, in which she tried to make her "transitional object." That was the time when we switched back to weekly sessions. Nadja seemed to be ready for that step and adjusted very well.

As we started with her final big project "the mermaid puppet" (Figure 3.54: "Mermaid," therapeutic puppet by Nadja, 13 years) we initiated termination, using a calendar as a means of countdown. Therefore, as we developed the body of this puppet we went through different stages of termination process together.

Nadja decided that the hands should be the first body part to be done. Although she never had tried the technique of 3-D-shaping with newspaper and tape, she showed amazing skills, and an extraordinary ambition. She wanted the hands to look real. Against my suggestions to keep it simple, she finally managed to make amazing expressive hands with long elegant fingers all on her own. Although we followed the countdown of the calendar during these sessions she seemed to be in absolute denial with the theme of termination.

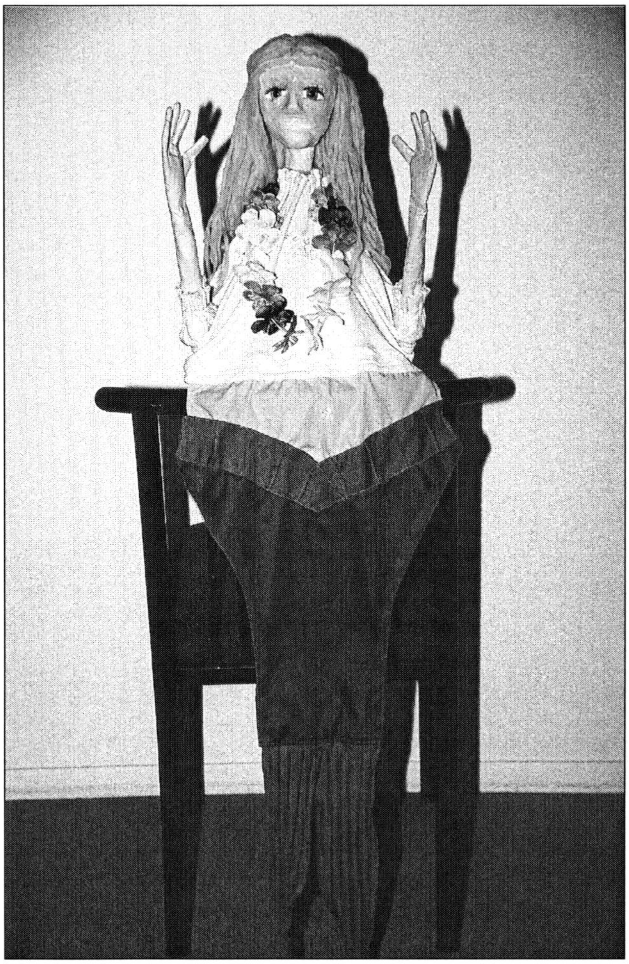

Figure 3.54. *Mermaid*, therapuetic puppet by Nadja, 13 years.

With the initiation of the head she suddenly showed a regressive behavior, trying to pass me more and more tasks with the excuse that it was too difficult for her, which sounded incredible after having observed her with the hands. I had a hard time to motivate her. Again, there was no way to verbalize the fact of termination. I was wondering how much her regressive behavior was a sign for her unconscious anger about termination, about me leaving her.

While we were working at the facial traits, including the forehead, eye sockets, nose, glass eyes and eyelids, she seemed to awake again and became very initiative in developing plans for the wig, the body which had to have a tail, and so on. While we were concentrating on work during the session, she was organizing stuff at home and each session would bring her newest acquisitions: red yarn for the wig, eyelashes made of real human hair, beads to put into the braids and to make a bracelet, and so on. During this stage the main theme was bargaining with termination. Now she started to ask about what I was doing after the art therapy program, and if there would be a possibility to keep me here. I disclosed to her about my plans of going back to medicine, hoping that one day I could be both a physician and an art therapist for sick children. So she started to make plans to look for a job for me, if not at a hospital possibly with her own pediatrician with whom she would arrange a meeting for me. Over and over again she told me that she would like me to become a doctor again, so that I would come back to be her art therapist later.

When it came to the final touch of the face with make-up and hairstyle, and in making a sewing pattern for the body, there was another theme arising: Body image, femininity and sex appeal. Again we spent a lot of time in mixing skin colors, cutting and adding hairs to the wig, accentuating the lips with a strong outline, and so forth. The most striking thing was the body she planned and had it completed by a neighbor: a Barbie-like slim figure, with a pink top, showing the belly button with a piece of skin and a wonderful green tail. Despite my concerns about this narrow body (it still was a puppet and Nadja should be able to put her arms inside to play with!) Nadja was absolutely enthusiastic about her beauty. During this time termination was not a big theme anymore. I had the feeling that with all the business Nadja developed she was regressing into the stage of denial and displacement again.

For the second last session before Nadja was allowed to take home her puppet, she brought a Hawaiian necklace made of artificial flowers for her puppet, "as a welcome sign at home." I had the strong feeling that by making the puppet as real-looking as possible Nadja tried to make a girlfriend for herself, or a substitute for me as a transitional object for her. This welcome ceremony demonstrated how much Nadja was able to identify with her puppet. Therefore, the puppet did not just represent a transitional object for her, but could function as an extension of Nadja and help her to express verbally things she would not dare to express personally.

At the end of this session we would have had enough time to enliven the mermaid puppet. I tried to engage the puppet in a verbal conversation, asking her how it would feel to leave the hospital and to go to a new home. Hoping to address the termination I let the puppet know, that with her leaving that day we would not be able to see each other anymore. But Nadja did not feel or was not ready to take over this role. Instead, she asked me to take a picture of her with the puppet and with Mr. Happy Potato Head she brought back for this occasion. On the one hand she simply was enjoying her puppet as a piece of art she accomplished, not yet being able to identify with her. On the other hand Nadja definitely wanted me to keep her in mind including all her favorite characters.

For weeks Nadja was planning to make her own dream catcher with me in her last session – something she could take home and would remind her of art therapy together with me (Figure 3.55: "My Dream Catcher," by Nadja, 13 years).

She wanted to make a star of rainbow-colored beads inside the dream catcher, and add a lot of purple and pink feathers (the colors of transition). It was our last teamwork, and together we added bead after bead. It reminded me of the rainbow and the rainbow-colored fence in her very first picture. An attempt for wholeness and perfection? Or the hope for a new beginning?

During this whole session termination was again the main theme. But this time she seemed to have accepted it. She was wondering if it would be possible to see me every once in a while, when I was working at the hospital; or if there was a possibility to keep in touch through the child life specialist, knowing that she would not get my address from the hospital or the unit. At the same time she was making plans for her own future, and was thinking about what she could do to shorten the dialysis time.

I started to work as a pediatrician at the department of Adolescent Medicine. One month later the staff doctor who is in charge for patients with planned transplantation approached me. Nadja was able to track me down, and to have her doctor prescribe art therapy in preparation for her transplantation. That was how we started to work together again. I was surprised about the developmental progress she made in the meantime.

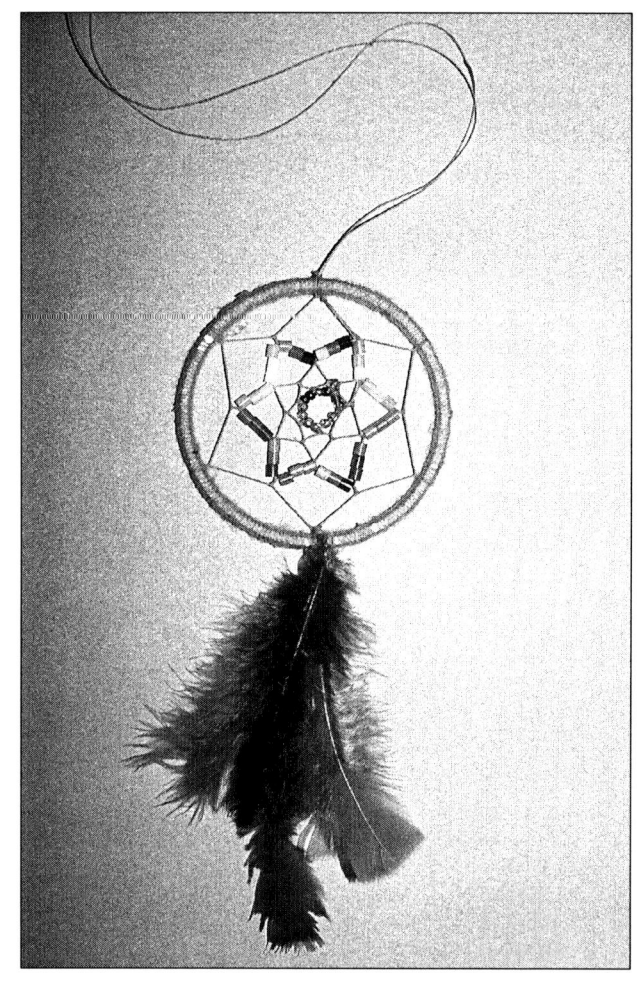

Figure 3.55. *My Dream Catcher*, by Nadja, 13 years.

SUMMARY

Thirteen-year-old Nadja was exceedingly able to connect with me. Loving art, she invested a lot into her artwork, using it to express and explore her inner struggle around body image, sexuality, and identity. Typically, she used her art in a metaphoric way, but without being ready to process it verbally. After having established a trustful working alliance, she started to show her true self with a high need for attention and of keeping control over the situation. Soon she would show her demanding and manipulative behavior, and we went through a period of time of pulling and pushing boundaries, very much like the two main characters in her mermaid story were doing. Finally, a calmer episode followed where she seemed to integrate her new acquaintances into her identity, in order to get ready for the next step of development.

Chapter 4

DISCUSSION

Patients with end-stage renal failure have high mortality and morbidity despite technological progress in hemodialysis, peritoneal dialysis and transplant procedures (Weldt, 2003).

> Children on dialysis face many problems directly attributable to their illness: body-image concerns, developmental delay, low self-esteem, anxiety, feelings of loss of control, dependency, and depression. . . . Children receiving dialysis leave normal life behind and enter a life of illness, recurrent hospitalization, and heightened vulnerability. (Wadeson, 2000, p. 129)

According to Meijer, chronic illness may interfere with the developmental tasks of adolescence by making the adolescent more vulnerable to psychological and social problems (2002). She states that there are both risk factors and resistance factors. The risk factors are disease/disability parameters, functional dependence and psychosocial stressors. The resistance factors include intrapersonal factors (e.g., temperament, problem-solving ability, etc.); socioeconomic factors (e.g., family environment, family member's adjustment, social support, etc.); and stress-processing factors (e.g., coping strategies, etc.) (Meijer, 2002). "Resistance factors are thought to moderate the negative effects of risk factors on psychosocial adjustment" (Meijer, 2002, p. 1453). Meijer found in her study that "psychosocial functioning of chronically ill adolescents was significantly related to stress-processing factors" (Meijer, 2002, p. 1459). According to her, stimulating functional coping styles may prevent developmental problems in psychosocial functioning. And this is where art therapy may play a significant role. Art therapy may be useful in stimulating functional coping styles in chronic physically ill adolescents by: (1) facilitating expression and understanding of emotions through artwork, ideally including verbal expression; (2) enhancing self-esteem and identity; and (3) offering an opportunity to vent anger and frustration (catharsis).

Making art appeared to enhance a positive attitude in patients and to give them feelings of power, control and freedom. It also seemed to provide patients with a sense of achievement. Even though the sessions I carried out were often interrupted by nurses who periodically checked blood pressure and dialysis machines, the participants were willing to carry on with their art projects and were able to concentrate on their work.

In working with an adolescent population it is important to understand the adolescent as an individual. One has to first try to understand the developmental stage of the individual, including the actual stage of life. Then one has to realize the importance of allowing the client to freely move from one developmental stage to another, with the therapist offering support and assistance. However, because of the individuality of the clients – and their respective past life experiences, cultural backgrounds and psychosocial issues (e.g., family dynamics, etc.) – it is impossible to make general assumptions about the extent of the effectiveness of art therapy in this population. In this chapter, therefore, I will explore this effectiveness on an individual basis. As Riley (1999) mentioned, "no two teenagers are on precisely the same path on maturation. I no longer evaluate the teen chronologically, I consider him or her developmentally" (p. 19).

Unlike Weldt (2003) in her study with adult hemodialysis patients (in which she offered well-defined directives), I decided to use spontaneous art with my population. By offering the teenagers the freedom to choose themes, materials and techniques, I hoped to provide them with a sense of empowerment and control – power and control being the biggest losses associated with any chronic physical illness. All of my clients, in one form or another, seemed to make use of this freedom. Even Jayson, who often exhibited defiant and rejective behavior, was attracted by it – so much so that, despite a period of crisis (due to difficulties in forming a trustful working alliance), whenever I offered him the opportunity to terminate the program, he refused. Instead, he chose to struggle through the entire nine-month period even though he knew his participation was voluntary. He seemed to like the fact that he was in control of the situation, or at least in control of this small part of his life. Another sign that he appreciated having control: the fact that it was up to him to set an end to his program, rather than going along with the fixed six-week termination time.

Like Wadeson (2000), I found spontaneous art to be more helpful in giving me an understanding of what the adolescents were experiencing, or what was important to them at any given point in time. I always kept some of the well-established directives (e.g., "My Tree," Bridge drawing) in the back of my mind in case the client asked for an idea of what to create. Although the majority of my clients would request an idea at some point, they rarely engaged in suggested directives. Only the older boys (Abdul, Martin) explored these directives; and only Abdul was able to gain some insight through doing these pieces. Of particular interest were his two bridge drawings, one made about six months before the other. It was fascinating to see how Abdul was able to express the different stages in his life before and after his kidney transplant. It was also fascinating to watch him gain insight through processing the pictures. Clearly, one needs some cognitive maturity to be able to process these kind of directed pictures.

Interestingly enough, none of my patients directly brought up the theme of disease or restriction in their spontaneous art. In contrast to Leonhard's (1984) findings in working with Cystic Fibrosis patients, I could not find typical features or drawing elements related to kidney disease. In the themes my population used, all dealt with the more general aspects of their lives, such as adolescence (e.g., body image, sexuality, independence, etc.) and psychosocial issues (e.g., fear of abandonment, feelings of isolation, family issues, etc.). Sometimes working on a specific piece of art triggered a verbal response about the disease, an occurrence that happened much more frequently and openly with clients in the late onset of the disease (Abdul, Katja, Nadja). Abdul and Nadja, for instance, often mentioned their disease, repeatedly telling me about their past experiences, but also talking to me about their futures, of what it will be like to live with their disease. In the group with early onset of the disease (Emma, Jayson, Joan, Martin), I found two reactions: they either avoided it (Jayson, Martin) or they totally integrated it into their lives (Emma, Joan). What can explain the different reactions between the genders? Perhaps the two girls simply were not conscious enough of their disease and physical restrictions to bring them up, or maybe for Emma and Joan they were just not an issue anymore, being part of their life experience. I am hesitant to make any conclusions about the avoidant behavior of the two boys. Was it related to gender, in the sense that males tend not to verbalize issues as much as females do? Or was it part of their overall lack of attachment to me as their therapist? In Jayson's case I wonder whether the avoidance was part of his resistance in the form of denial. Since Jayson and his family were never able to mourn and accept their father's death, perhaps the family was not able to accept Jayson's physical illness either.

At this point in the chapter I will explore the effectiveness of art therapy in my population, starting with the short-term group, followed by the long-term group. An important factor in considering the potential effectiveness of art therapy is the duration of a client's participation in the program. My experience is that it takes the client between five to twelve sessions to finally let the mask fall and to be more open. That is what Moon (1998) calls "the initial phase of resistance," in which the partners of a treatment program work on developing a "working alliance." Since the adolescents in the short-term group only worked with me for a limited number of sessions (between five and eleven), I am hesitant to consider these sessions as therapeutic, particularly because they were not directed nor insight-oriented. (It is possible to lead short-term, insight-oriented art therapy treatments, but only with limited goals and well-defined, goal-focused directives in a mature population) (Wadeson, 1980).

I consider a patient contact to be "therapeutic" if the client was able to begin to develop awareness of underlying issues, to begin to work through conflicts, and to start developing problem-solving strategies and coping styles. However, perhaps my standards for "therapeutic" may be too high. Potentially even one session could have some limited therapeutic value. With my teenagers in the short-term group we never went beyond the initial phase of resistance. Although all were able to identify – and express – a variety of issues through their art, I never had the feeling that any of them were deeply conscious of what they had raised. Nor were any of these teens ready to confront the issues before them. Therefore, I am hesitant to make any statements about therapeutic effects of art therapy in these short-term cases. However, it is possible that by simply expressing the issues in their art and by developing their relationship with me there was indeed some therapeutic impact.

Discussion

For all human beings, it takes time to develop a "trustful working alliance." If one meets a person once a week, as in this kind of therapeutic setting, it may take weeks to establish enough mutual trust and confidence before a client opens up. Therefore, in my short-term group the limitation was the lack of a "trustful working alliance." In two cases, that of Emma and Martin, we did not have enough time to establish a deeper working alliance during their hospitalization, or to help them bridge the gap of discharge from hospital. I wonder if they would have continued art therapy on an out-patient basis if we did have enough time to know and trust each other more profoundly. Joan's case is different. She was referred to art therapy only towards the end of the program and, therefore, the benefit of the art-making process was limited.

As I mentioned in a previous chapter, Moon (1998) observed different types of resistances. Emma, for instance, was a good example of resistance through "compliant surrender." As well, by exhibiting very controlled behavior similar to that of an adult, she also showed some typical defense mechanisms for her age group (Neinstein, 1991; Hofmann, 1997; Linesch, 1988). The defense mechanisms were:

1. *Intellectualization*; e.g., she had rational explanations about her disease and treatment, and was perfectly able to suppress her emotions about that topic at the same time;
2. *Displacement*; e.g., she displaced all feelings concerning her neediness for emotional nourishment and support, which were expressed in a metaphoric way in all her art pieces and in her efforts to connect with me;
3. *Isolation*; e.g., in her questions around the hemodialysis unit and about my work with the children there, she detached her feelings of being separated, excluded and abandoned from the actual content of her concern; and finally
4. *Denial*, which is based on my speculation; e.g., denial of her loneliness and neediness for support and emotional nourishment, which were expressed in her art work, her serious efforts to connect with me, and her obvious disappointment regarding peer contact on the hemodialysis unit, and so forth – all of which made me suspicious about the truth of what she told me of her social environment. Her story about a lot of good friends at school, for example, seemed to be a form of denial of a social isolation rather than reality.

Martin, on the other hand, was a good example of resistance through "running away." With his shy and withdrawn behavior he demonstrated some typical defense mechanisms. They were:

1. *Intellectualization*; e.g., through his rational explanation of his soldier models, stressing his interest in history, he was able to disguise his unconscious anger and aggression.
2. *Isolation*; e.g., he was able to detach and repress his own underlying feelings of anger and aggression from the actual content of his creative activity (war objects).
3. *Regression*; e.g., the only way to get the attention he needed was to become the baby of the family, especially to his grandmother.
4. *Denial*; e.g., whenever I brought up the theme of his physical condition and the surgical intervention, he reacted with avoidance, withdrawal or immediately changed the subject.
5. *Reversal of affect*; e.g., sibling rivalry seemed to be a real conflict for him, but whenever negative feelings towards his brother came up, he turned them into admiration for his brother.

Martin's vulnerability and lack of grounding were metaphorically reflected in his rootless, free-floating tree and in his unstable bridge. The fact that he was dependent on detailed construction plans – in other words, on a lot of support for his creative activity – reinforced these observations. His shy, withdrawn and sometimes avoidant behavior were the results of low self-esteem and poor self-confidence, perhaps partly due to living in the shadow of a dominant brother.

In this context Joan's case seems to be more difficult. Due to her severe congenital malformation syndrome, Joan seemed to be a good example of an individual who had managed to integrate her physical impairment into her identity and to achieve satisfactory adaptation (Hofmann, 1997). The support of her social environment was crucial for this development. On the one hand I never felt any kind of direct resistance with her; in fact, I rather sensed her gratitude for whoever was willing to spend some time with her and whoever was interested in what she had to tell. On the other hand, though, one could argue that she was another typical case of resistance through "compliant surrender" – her main defense mechanisms being displacement and denial. However, I have not had evidence to confirm this.

Therefore, with the population of the short-term group it would be difficult in my opinion to make speculations about the therapeutic effectiveness of art therapy due the early point at which we had to stop the program. Although these short-term treatments may have had limited therapeutic value, there were some gains in identifying issues and conflicts by giving initial permission to express them. Thus, these advances may be considered to be a positive effect of art therapy in short-term treatments. As well, the patients may have benefited from their relationship with me. Just by having someone listen to them and support them in a non-judgmental way may have been helpful in allowing them to take further developmental steps. After coming to an understanding of some of the issues involved in these particular cases, I am convinced that the adolescents would have benefited from art therapy after they had established a trustful working alliance.

To explore the effectiveness of art therapy in the population of the long-term group I used Erikson's Psychosocial theory for a developmental staging, and an Object-Relations approach to describe the therapeutic process. The summarized tasks characterizing the developmental stage of the adolescent are: (1) achieving independence from parents; (2) adopting peer codes and life styles; (3) becoming aware of the importance of body image and of acceptance of one's body image; and finally (4) establishing sexual, ego, vocational and moral identities (Neinstein, 1991). Two out of four clients were able to develop some independence from their parents: Abdul started to spend more of his spare time outside his family and to invest in relationships with peers; and Nadja successfully participated and had fun in summer camp for kidney patients. Therefore, both were more able to explore and adopt peer lifestyles. They both were able to use art as a starting point with which to discuss and work through identity issues. The same two clients seemed to become aware of the importance of their body image, and explored and exercised its acceptance, including sexuality. However, with the kind of chronic physical illness my population suffered from, I would expect a resolution of their body-image issues to be a lifelong process. Finally, one out of four clients started to establish some sexual, vocational and moral identity. Abdul, as the oldest of my long-term clients, started to make some concrete educational plans in order to reach his high professional goal of becoming a lawyer. He not only explored moral issues in his art, but we often had interesting discussions in which we compared different religious and moral points of view. By contrast, in the case of Jayson and Katja, they couldn't possibly embrace adolescent issues in a positive way until they first solved big issues that were rooted in earlier developmental stages.

In general, three out of four teens coped better at the end of the art therapy program than they did at the start. They improved their capacities to make decisions, taking over control and responsibility in treatment, and performing flexibility and strength through improvisations in coping with their disease. Only one seemed not to have significantly changed his behavior by the end of the program, keeping up his particular pattern of defensive behavior for the entire nine months.

Katja, at 12 years of age, was my youngest female client in the long-term group. According to Erikson (1968) she was in the developmental stage of "Identity vs. Role Confusion." As far as I understood, based on what Katja's father told me of her history, she went through a normal early childhood, together with her sister, who was two years older, and her younger brother, who was six years younger. Thanks to the engagement, the consistency and continuity of her parents, particularly her father, she developed a basic capacity for trust and a rudimentary sense of ego-identity. However, she always exhibited a shy, quiet and withdrawn temperament; therefore, she always seemed to have had a hard time holding her own ground towards her temperamentally and physically stronger sister. I think that sibling dynamics need to be kept in mind when considering Katja's development during the stage of "Autonomy vs. Shame and Doubt." In this stage, when Katja was confronted with her first boundary issues, she probably had to give up a lot of privacy, in favor of her sister's privacy, despite their parents' interventions in holding back the sister. Therefore, Katja never learned to keep rivals out, but would rather withdraw and leave the "battlefield." At the end of Erikson's stage of "Industry vs. Inferiority," Katja was attacked by a terrible illness, leaving big scars not only in a physical sense, but in a psychological sense as well. This girl, who had already developed doubts and inferiority feelings in her ego-identity, suffered a significant regression. Her father confirmed my assumption: that through this disease Katja had lost a good part of her already low self-confidence and self-esteem. When entering "Early Adolescence" (Golombek et al., 1989), Katja had to deal again with challenges of her early childhood. The stress of the new physical and psychosocial changes that overtook her was increased at least twofold by her existing physical conditions, which made her even more vulnerable and anxious. Her reaction was to withdraw and to mistrust people – and that was how she was when I met her. She only had a few people she trusted.

Discussion

At the beginning of the nine-month art therapy program it took us a few sessions to form a trustful working alliance. During this initial phase of resistance, according to Moon (1998), Katja did not dare to talk to me on her own. I would consider her to be an example of resistance through "running away." The way she needed her child-life specialist to transfer her replies and wishes to me, the way she initially avoided me were both forms of running away. However, after we did form that trustful working alliance, she did not need the child-life specialist anymore. The defense mechanisms typical for her during the program were:

1. *Regression*; e.g., although she was compliant in a medical sense, she avoided taking over small responsibilities, even in the art-making process, and moved back to a more child-like dependence, asking me to make decisions for her.
2. *Denial*; e.g., threatening aspects of the disease were suppressed, as if they were non-existing.
3. *Displacement*; e.g., she tended to substitute concerns about herself with concerns about, primarily, her sister, but about her father as well.
4. *Isolation*; e.g., in some of her art pieces she demonstrated the separation of her emotions from the actual content of the piece of art (aggression or fear in the case of the bee family).

In general, she loved to do arts and crafts, and seemed content with our working relationship. Her main issue was to gain self-confidence and enhance her self-esteem. From an object relations perspective (St. Clair, 2000), she needed first to internalize some successful relationships with good objects in order to develop a healthy independence. On the one hand I got a strong feeling of the weakness of her "true self," and the development of her "false self." She showed a strong tendency to suppress her own individuality and to mold herself to the needs of others, mainly her sister. Therefore, she was overly compliant. But on the other hand I sensed her very strong attachment to me, after she was able to trust me, as her object. In her regression she appeared to be back in the early emotional stage, at which a close attachment and physical consistent presence are important. An obvious sign of her regression was her use of clay, the material with which she appeared to be most comfortable at that early stage of treatment. (Clay with its muddy softness and moisture is often used by children in early developmental stages or in phases of regression) (Wadeson, 1987). At the time of treatment she seemed to need me as her "auxiliary ego" as part of her process in developing a sense of self, which showed itself when, following a few weeks of developing some security through the use of clay, she indicated that she was ready to switch to the more progressive technique of drawing, initially sticking with the more controllable crayons. In a metaphoric sense, she needed my outline drawings to be contained, and to feel safe during the exploration of her own individuality. In this context I wonder whether her art could be considered to be a kind of "transitional object," which would explain her need to take home her clay objects as soon as possible. The more security she gained, it seemed, the more she was able to switch to less controllable techniques like pastels, or even watercolors, which was another sign of her progressing development. Step-by-step she took over the outline drawing, initially by copying my drawings that had been made on a separate piece of paper, and then later by developing her own shapes.

In summary, her extreme physical dependence induced a remarkable developmental regression in an emotional sense, which resulted in an almost symbiotic relationship with me as her therapist. Therefore, for the whole duration of art therapy with Katja I observed that few adolescent issues arose. She obviously had to first deal with earlier issues. However, in my opinion she definitely benefited from art therapy, particularly when one compares her initial insecurity to the increased autonomy she had gained by the end of the program. Through her therapy she gained some self-confidence and enhanced her self-esteem.

Although Jayson and Nadja were about the same age, they had totally different responses to art therapy. Despite sharing similar religious and cultural backgrounds, their previous life experiences had been very different. Jayson had a big psychosocial burden (death of his father, etc.) to bear on top of the early onset of his disease. By contrast, Nadja, as a result of the late onset of her disease, enjoyed a relatively stable psychosocial environment. I will explore their responses to art therapy individually.

Jayson, at 13 years of age, was my youngest male client in the long-term group. According to Erikson (1968), he was in the developmental stage of "Identity vs. Role Confusion." According to Golombek et al. (1989), he was in "Early Adolescence," in which the child is dealing again with early challenges that root in Erikson's (1968) stage of "Trust vs. Mistrust." According to Jones, an "individual recapitulates and expands in the second decennium of life the development he passed through during the first five years" (Anna Freud, 1958, p. 256). He postulated that "adolescence recapitulates infancy" (Anna Freud, 1958, p. 256).

During therapy Jayson behaved like a child who had never had a chance to experience a reliable "holding environment," something necessary in order to develop a healthy self-esteem and the capability of self-containment one would expect of a 13-year-old adolescent. I consider both, a healthy self-esteem and the capability for self-containment, crucial for compliance in a medical sense. How could Jayson possibly show therapeutic compliance for his physical conditions without having a sense of self-worth and enough self-confidence? It was not, however, entirely clear whether Jayson had regressed as a result of his illness and the onset of adolescence, or whether he never had a secure sense of self.

Nine months of art therapy with Jayson was characterized by short episodes of close work, interrupted by rejection and avoidance due to resistance. According to Moon (1998), he is an example of resistance through "running away," avoiding confrontation by non-participation. His typical defense mechanisms were:

1. *Denial*; e.g., threatening aspects of his disease or of his past life were suppressed, as if they did not exist.
2. *Isolation*; e.g., in his artwork he often separated his emotions from the content of his project (e.g., in Michael Jackson's glove he isolated his own feelings of vulnerability and helplessness from the content of admiration of a hero).
3. *Projection*; e.g., self-blame and guilt over a situation were often shifted to something or somebody else (e.g., his venous line).

As his art therapist I never really got the feeling that we had formed a close, reliable and trustful working alliance. Nor did I get the feeling that a secure attachment had been formed. I would rather consider Jayson's attachment to be insecure, with a disorganized coping style (Biringen, 1994). He showed the typical fluctuation in attachment strategies, which included tense proximity-seeking followed by intense avoidance and displays of simultaneous contradictory behavior patterns, such as ignoring me while working with me. He never was able to create a secure attachment that would provide him with a secure base from which he could have explored both self and others.

His physical problems started at the age of 5, an age at which the awareness of bodily integrity is crucial for the development of a healthy body image. His damaged body image, together with a potential lack of secure attachment, perhaps led to reduced self-worth and self-confidence. Due to his lack of ego-strength, he developed a "false self," which kept feelings of a hidden "true self" from arising. Fearing unbearable failures, he was neither ready for explorations, nor for taking risks, nor for trials. Often when he did not feel physically well enough to do art, I had the impression that he was not physically strong enough to keep the feelings under control. He then would refuse to do art, fearing the arousal of unbearable feelings – especially in context with the lack of sense for containment.

Considering this insecure attachment dynamic within the therapeutic setting, I wondered about Jayson's experience with his own mother during his early childhood. I have to make speculations, since his mother showed the same avoidance towards me as her son did, and therefore, I was never able to meet and get to know her. I doubt that his mother's emotional availability enabled Jayson "to venture away from her as well as refuel with her" (Biringen, 1994, p. 408). With the early onset of his physical illness he might have had an even higher need for a "holding environment" and "good enough mother" in Winnicott's sense (St. Clair, 2000).

Jayson's lack of motivation, his lack of investment into his art and his lack of interest in playing an active role in his life together with a deep underlying sadness and hopelessness were symptoms of his depression.

Often his non-compliance in medical treatment would lead to increased physical pain. Jayson's behavior often reminded me of the tendencies often observed in abuse victims – self-punishment or victimization based on a lack of self-worth or even on self-hate – it also reminded me of the chronic suicide attempts of deeply depressed people.

Maybe his non-compliance also had a component of "denial," "anger," "bargaining," and "depression" in Kuebler-Ross' terms (Kuebler-Ross, 1969–1997). Because Jayson and his family never were able to mourn and accept their father's death, maybe they were not able to accept Jayson's physical illness either.

I consider his reluctance to continue art therapy through to the termination period of six weeks to be his own all-too-soon termination. Based on an insecure attachment, the termination of art therapy for Jayson was comparable to abandonment, as his father had abandoned him. Since termination seemed to be too painful for him, perhaps he preferred to abandon me.

Through his art and his behavior as a result of insecure attachment, he showed his need to be allowed to be a child and to experience fundamental basics of containment without having to take over the burden of too much responsibility before he would have to confront further adolescent issues.

In summary, I believe that even Jayson, with his often defiant and rejective behavior, found some sort of benefit in art therapy. Because of his psychosocial issues it was a significant experience for him to get the feeling of his therapist's availability and consistent presence in a non-judgmental way, despite his ambivalent attitude. It was also important for him to gain a sense of mastery and control within his limited environment, so he could enhance his self-esteem. Finally, as Jayson confirmed verbally in his final session, it was important for him to have a distraction, to be allowed to move into a different world without disease and responsibility at least for a short time – and to have a forum in which the possibility of venting his feelings was possible.

However, Jayson's behavior and attitude throughout art therapy did not significantly change. His lack of motivation, his refusal to accept his disease, and his unwillingness to respond to his treatment prevailed. In addition, he still would not deal with his traumatic past. He entered adolescence with no reliable support system or stable parental figures. When I read Raghuraman's (2000) article, I found a lot of parallels between her client and mine. I wonder, that with enough time and more intensive treatment, if Jayson would have been able to eventually connect with me, in order to rehabilitate his internalization of a "good enough mother" and a "holding environment." However, I am convinced that to help Jayson, the investment and engagement in family therapy would be crucial.

Although Nadja was the same age as Jayson, her response to art therapy was quite different. According to Erikson (1968), she was in the developmental stage of "Identity vs. Role Confusion," and according to Golombek et al. (1989) she was in "Early Adolescence," in which the child is dealing again with early challenges that root in Erikson's (1968) stage of "Trust vs. Mistrust." She was referred to me because of her "highly demanding and manipulative behavior as symptoms of a secondary gain due to her chronic physical illness." The longer I was able to observe the almost symbiotic, and at the same time mutually controlling mother-daughter relationship, the more I understood that Nadja's behavior had little, if anything, to do with secondary gain of her physical illness – particularly if one keeps in mind that the control battle around food had already started in her early childhood. Nadja's behavior was more of a mirroring of the internalized controlling behavior of her overly responsible and protective mother. I considered Nadja's mother to be a very conscientious and overprotective person, someone who had a hard time giving up or sharing responsibility. I could imagine that this was the result of having had to deal on her own (i.e., without family support) first with a preterm baby and his problems, and then later with Nadja's severe physical illness. As a result, however, she seemed to find it difficult to either pass some responsibility over to Nadja or to let her take control over her life to a certain degree. Obviously, this problem went back to Nadja's early childhood (oral/anal stage) when food and eating habits became a power-control struggle for the first time. Due to her mother's reliability, Nadja showed an exemplary compliance in treatment, but due to her mother's control, she didn't seem to make decisions about her own friends, which led to social isolation. I consider her mother's reluctance to be tested as potential organ donor as a sign of her difficulties in giving up control. How could she possibly care full-time for Nadja if her own physical state was compromised?

According to Winnicott (1956), a flexible and genuine attachment with a "good enough mother" is essential to nurture the "true self." If a child has to be attuned to the needs of the caregiver, and/or his "holding environment" is overly limiting, he will develop a "false self." Therefore, Nadja's reaction was to develop a demanding behavior so her mother would be kept busy focusing on her. Although she ate only very little and highly selected items only, she liked to keep her mother busy exploring and inventing new recipes. Therefore, Nadja fulfilled her mother's need to care for her and protect her, which in turn would give her mother a meaningful life.

Over time Nadja and I were able to develop a trustful working alliance, one that included her mother, with whom I was in regular contact. Because of this relationship, Nadja's mother was able to give up her control to some extent and transfer some of the responsibility for her daughter onto me, which helped the two of them to establish a more relaxed relationship, leaving more private space to each other.

Nadja's development during seven months of the art therapy program can be subdivided in four stages:

Stage one: Building a trustful working alliance: Moon (1998) calls this initial phase "resistance." Nadja would fit his definition for a resistance through "compliant surrender." Trying to fulfill my potential expectations she mobilized her whole range of aesthetic perfection in her art (e.g., colorful rainbows, flowers, decorative garlands, etc.).

After getting to know each other and becoming attuned, Nadja increasingly lost the facade of the nice, cooperative "good girl." Step-by-step, her true self emerged, showing a controlling-commanding and manipulative behavior towards me that she apparently used to show towards her mother. Perhaps in seeing me as her transferential mother she was testing my boundaries, to see how far I would tolerate exploitation. As soon as I made a comment on that matter, her reaction was withdrawal in passive aggression and defiance. With respect of her personal safety, I let her take control over the session as much as possible. I even allowed her to eat during the session in order to avoid the power-control struggle over food.

Nadja's range of characteristic defense mechanisms included:

1. *Intellectualization*; e.g., when suppressing the emotional part of an issue, she tended to deal with it with rational objectivity, offering an interesting range of rational explanations.
2. *Regression*; e.g., in order to avoid unbearable responsibilities, she moved back to child-like dependence.
3. *Projection*; e.g., when encountering self-blame or guilt over a situation, she often shifted her emotions onto her mother.
4. *Displacement*; e.g., often she replaced concerns about herself with concerns about her mother.
5. *Compensation*; e.g., with her highly developed creativity she was able to replace lost or missed qualities by new constructed activities.

I wonder if Nadja's controlling behavior and need for perfection were symptoms of feeling vulnerable and helpless, and fear that she really cannot manage on her own.

Stage two: Exploring adolescent issues: During this stage, Nadja's behavior toward me changed almost from one session to the next. She did not command me anymore, but rather included me in her working process as an attentive listener to her story or as her art therapist. Our teamwork changed from a commander-worker relationship to a more explorer-assistant relationship. My main task was to offer her the "holding environment," in which she could facilitate explorations of adolescent issues. By designing the so adverse characters of the two mermaids, including their mothers as exaggeration, Nadja created an ideal stage on which to explore issues of identity, body image and sexuality, independence and peer relationships, including jealousy and rivalry. The underwater world provided a safe environment in which to express the conflictual and darker side of herself and her relationships.

During this time, her mother played a more passive role and often withdrew to read a book.

Stage three: Food and eating habits as weapons in control struggle: I was surprised when I got the news about the G-tube implantation. Apparently Nadja had reached a critical level of weight loss that made medical intervention necessary. At the same time, Nadja had started another major project – Mr. Happy Potato Head as a papier maché bowl with a big mouth to store and offer lots of candies to whoever deserved them. Since early childhood, food and eating habits apparently were the battlefields for control issues between mother and daughter. By getting this G-tube, which made it possible to infuse high-caloric formula while sleeping, Nadja lost the last possibility of keeping control. But by designing this bowl for candies she symbolically created another means of control of this oral issue. On the one hand, the papier maché bowl seemed to reflect Nadja's enormous need to be nurtured and fed. On the other hand, though, the bowl also provided for others, so, perhaps, she wouldn't appear to be like a greedy child, not willing to let go. During this stage the processing of her actual issues was more on a verbal basis, while she was performing the monotonous task of gluing layers and layers of newspaper, controlling her own pace. By choosing the technique of the messiness of papier maché (which, similar to clay, is a sign for regression (Wadeson, 1987), she definitively went back to the oral (nurturing) and anal (controlling) stage, trying to get back the control she might have missed in her early childhood. Interestingly enough, during this period of time, her mother again played a more active, controlling role. Due to the surgical intervention and her task to infuse the formula at night time, her instinct for responsibility and over-protectiveness seemed to have reawakened, which intensified Nadja's endeavor for exploration.

Stage four: Exploring body image and making a transitional object: The beginning of Nadja's last major project coincided with the initiation of the termination process. While we were elaborating on the facial and bodily feature of her mermaid puppet, the main verbal theme was termination. The stages we went through reminded me of Kuebler-Ross' stages of acceptance of death (Kuebler-Ross, 1969) – denial, anger, bargaining, and, finally, acceptance. Through all these stages, there were episodes of sadness and regression.

By choosing the mermaid as her theme again, Nadja symbolized her need to go back to the search for her identity, as she did in her mermaid story. Through this mermaid, she got a wonderful opportunity to explore body image and sex appeal as parts of her identity. If she was to explore feelings about sexuality, there was no way to address it, similar to stage two, when she was dealing with these issues through the metaphor of her mermaid story. The reason may have been partly her reluctance, but for sure the lack of confidentiality in this non-ideal setting. I had the feeling that, by making her puppet look as real as possible, Nadja was trying to create a girlfriend for herself, or a substitute for me, like a transitional object. In Nadja's case, this puppet not only gave her a permanent figure which she could use to express herself verbally without being personally involved, it also provided her with an object that she could fully control.

In summary, by the use of art therapy as a "holding environment" Nadja was able to work on adolescent struggles regarding self-identification, self-differentiation, and separation in a metaphorical (through telling stories) and symbolic (the mermaid as her self-representation) way. At the same time she was able to discuss and work through other issues with roots in earlier developmental stages (feeding/control issues). Her transference towards me seemed to change from an initial maternal transference with power/control issues into a more collegial one, which gave her the opportunity to check out different lifestyles and opinions.

My fourth long-term client, Abdul at 16 years, was the oldest. According to Erikson (1968), he was in the developmental stage of "Identity vs. Role Confusion," and according to Golombek et al.

(1989) he was in "Late Adolescence," in which the adolescent has to face again challenges associated with Erikson's (1968) stage of "Initiative vs. Guilt." With an increased ability to be introspective, the child appears to be more willing to attempt to influence his environment.

Thanks perhaps in part to a more healthy and supportive family dynamic, Abdul was able to develop a pretty stable identity structure. However, with his chronic physical illness with late onset at the age of 15, which most likely provoked his family to leave India, he had to face a new aspect of identity crisis.

As his art therapist I had the good fortune to accompany Abdul through his nine months of transition. The program started when he was still on hemodialysis, continued through intense verbal therapy while he was an inpatient for transplantation, and, finally, it assisted him in exploring his new life until just before he was released from hospital treatment. Abdul's development during nine months of art therapy could be subdivided in four stages:

Stage one: Forming a trustful working relationship: While keeping his feelings tamed by defense mechanisms of politeness and aesthetics, Abdul was able to relate and connect with me, and introduced me into his world of an immigrant and chronic physically ill adolescent. According to Moon (1998), at this stage Abdul, with his politeness and overadaptability, was a good example of resistance through "compliant surrender." His range of characteristic defense mechanisms included:

1. *Intellectualization*; e.g., suppressing the emotional part of an issue, he tended to deal with it in a more objective way by offering interesting rational explanations.
2. *Compensation*; e.g., due to his highly developed curiosity and above average intelligence he was able to replace lost qualities by new constructive activities, like literature searches and acquisition of new knowledge (e.g., archeology, etc.).
3. *Denial*; e.g., he tended to suppress threatening aspects of an issue, as if they did not exist.
4. *Projection*; e.g., he often shifted self-blame and guilt over a situation onto something else (e.g., school problems, foreign cultural environment, etc.).

Stage two: Adolescent defiance and struggle for independence: The more that trust was established, the more Abdul allowed himself to lift the curtain of defense and show his true self. During this period of persistent portrait drawing and moving within a very narrow range of themes, Abdul was even less spontaneous in his artistic expression. But he seemed to be much more genuine in his behavior, showing his passive aggressive traits towards me. According to Moon (1998), in this stage Abdul switched to the resistance group of "I'm in the In-crowd/You're in the Out-crowd." The fact of his defiant-rejective behavior towards me, in comparison to his flirtatious behavior with the nurses, brought up questions about his transference. In his attempt to search for his identity and push its development, he fought for independence. In this struggle for independence he was obviously fighting against his transferential authority, control figure as part of the health care system, and of the parental figure I represented to him. But he also showed typical adolescent behavior, pulled and pushed by his own ambivalence of feelings between love and hate. For him, it was much safer to go through this battle with me in the "holding environment" of art therapy than to struggle with his parents who he was dependent on because of his illness and his unconscious fear of abandonment. He could not dare to show his parents his anger and defiance because they had already sacrificed a lot for his own sake, and he would still be dependent on them for a long time. That was why he made use of me as the temporary replacement of a "good enough mother." Remembering my own countertransference during this stage, I wondered how far I witnessed "projective identification." Did he feel himself rejected and excluded from life, like I felt excluded from having fun with the nurses? The reason for the difference in the way he treated the nurses and myself perhaps he had connected with me on a deeper emotional level, which increased the risk of a potential dependence. At the same time, he had to behave with the nurses, because he still might be dependent on their goodwill for a long time.

His flirtatious behavior with the nurses during this phase may also have been his way of dealing with, and exploring feelings about, sexuality. However, whenever I made a comment about his behavior, or I tried to address it, I encountered denial. In his own words, it was just my interpretation. As there was no way to address his behavior, there was no way to address this issue either, in part due to his reluctance (because I was female?), and in part because of the non-ideal setting, with its lack of confidentiality.

But, as with a "good enough mother," he had an opportunity to experience my unconditional care, despite his rejection. Slowly he was ready to change his transference towards me from a parental into a peer figure.

Stage three: Regression through physical invasion: Due to the intense physical invasion of the kidney transplantation, he showed a remarkable regression. His well-functioning family system became even more supportive and empathetic after transplantation. Having the loving care of both parents, his transference towards me switched to a needed peer figure. After having achieved a certain degree of independence, he now needed to test and adopt peer codes and lifestyles, to explore and form new relationships with objects of his new cultural environment. As his art therapist, I accompanied him on his journey of discovery through this new world.

Stage four: Exploring the future: Through previous developmental stages, Abdul was able to come to a place of identification and separateness at the same time. With me as his art therapist he was able to relieve his burden by sharing his responsibility. Through its consistency and safety, art therapy represented a "holding environment" within the turbulence of Abdul's new life after transplantation, this being a difficult time of transition between hospital/medical life and the outside world. Now he was ready to use art as an extension of his own restricted world and explore his future and gain control of his life.

In summary, through the use of art therapy as a "holding environment," one that included a needed object on which to rely on, Abdul was able to discuss and to re-establish his identity structure. Thanks to his artistic engagement in visual expression and highly developed curiosity, he was able to gain a fair amount of insight by processing (mainly directed) art projects verbally. Through his initial defiant behavior towards me as his transferential mother, he gained a sense of independence and control over his life, which helped him to overcome the short period of regression during surgery. His later behavior towards me was more like a peer with whom he shared experiences, explored different lifestyles and moral issues, although he remained reluctant in dealing more openly with sexuality. He was able to integrate newly discovered aspects of his new cultural environment into his personality, and, finally, started to explore professional possibilities for his future life, including ego, vocational and moral identities. Over time he was able to develop good relationships with peers. He started to replace me as his transferential peer with true friends, and to develop an active social life outside of his family. During the last few sessions of the art therapy program he did not feel like drawing anymore. Instead, he used them to wrap up and share with me his smaller and bigger successes in life, including his education, social life and illness. Of all my patients, Abdul's termination was the only one that I truly felt was appropriate.

SUMMARY

By reviewing the long-term population's responses to art therapy, I found that all four clients benefited from this experience in their own particular way. For Abdul and Nadja, who were lucky enough to have the support of relatively healthy family dynamics, this was the opportunity to deal with adolescent issues without jeopardizing their relationship with their supporting objects. For Jayson and Katja, who had to deal with remarkable challenges with roots back in their early childhood, it was more about recapitulating early developmental stages in order to make up for the missed parts of development. According to Anna Freud (1958), they both would have to face and work through these early issues first, before they would be able to embrace adolescent issues connected with their developmental age. In every case but Abdul's, I definitely felt that termination, although started ahead of time – that it would last 6 weeks – was artificial and inappropriate. However, all four benefited from art therapy, though each could have benefited from longer-term work.

It is my belief that if the environment in which I was working had been more supportive and open-minded, even greater success could have been achieved.

CONCLUSION

It is important to focus on the limitations of this study in order to plan additional studies to further explore the effectiveness of art therapy for a population of adolescents with chronic physical ailments.

The biggest limitation to this study was the far from ideal setting, where it was impossible to work in a one-to-one situation with the client. Due to the presence of other children on hemodialysis, and the necessary interruptions of the session by the nurses who had to check the patient's vital signs and the machine on a regular basis, confidentiality could not be guaranteed. This made it impossible to express and discuss difficult issues like sexuality, and so forth more openly, which definitely had a negative impact on the overall treatment of this adolescent population.

Finally, the limited time of nine months could also be considered a limitation of this study. In some cases (e.g., Jayson) the duration of the treatment of nine months may have been too short. As adolescents, they may need longer-term work. The duration of the therapy in this study may be just a beginning, especially with this kind of chronic physical illness, which causes a lot of interruptions of the treatment program.

Because this study dealt with a small number of patients, it is based more on a comparison of case studies. To make more general statements possible, a bigger and more diverse population would be necessary. Further studies with a bigger population, a broader spectrum of more diverse chronic physical diseases, and a higher age range within the developmental stage of adolescence are necessary.

For this study I reviewed the client's art and my own notes without using objective measures. Psychological assessments or other standardized objective measures before and after art therapy treatment could add significant information and underline my statements with more hard facts.

However, it is my belief that with this study I was able to prove that art therapy has had a positive effect on these chronic physically ill adolescents in dealing with personal and developmental issues.

I hope that with this work I was able to sensitize the people who have to deal with adolescents with a chronic physical illness, and to add to their understanding of these teenagers' potential issues and needs. Finally, I hope that I was able to demonstrate that as a worker in a health care facility we are all able to change the life of these adolescents, only by offering them appropriate empathy.

BIBLIOGRAPHY

Bach, S. (1995). *Life paints its own span.* Einsiedeln: Daimon Verlag.

Berzoff, J. (1996). Psychosocial ego development: The theory of Erk Erikson. In J. Berzoff, L.M. Flanagan & P. Hertz (Eds.), *Inside out and outside in,* 103–125. Northvale NJ: Jason Aronson, Inc.

Biringen, Z. (1994). Attachment theory and research: Application to clinical practice. *American Journal of Orthopsychiatry 64*(3), 404–418.

Blum, R. Wm. (1992), Chronic illness and disability in adolescence. *Journal of Adolescent Health, 13,* 364–368.

Boice, M.M. (1998). Chronic illness in adolescence. *Adolescence 33*(132), 927–939.

Boland, K. (1977). *Assessing personality through tree drawings.* New York: Basic Books, Inc., Publisher.

Buchanan, D.C. & Abram, H.S. (1984). Psychological Adaptation to Hemodialysis. In R.H. Moos (Ed.), *Coping with physical illness 2: New perspectives,* 273–281. New York: Plenum.

Cappelli, M. et al. (1989). Chronic disease and its impact. *Journal of Adolescent Health Care, 10,* 283–288.

Councill, T. (1993). Art therapy with pediatric cancer patients: Helping normal children cope with abnormal circumstances. *Art Therapy 10*(2), 78–87.

Edwards, M. (1987). Jungian Analytic Art Therapy. In J.A. Rubin (Ed.), *Approaches to art therapy: Theory and technique.* 92–133. Bristol, PA: Brunner/Mazel.

Eiser, Ch. (1993). *Growing up with a chronic disease.* London and Bristol, PA: Jessica Kingsley, Publishers.

Ellis, C.R. (2002). Eating disorder: Pica. Internet information: www.emedicine.com

Erikson, E. (1950/1963). *Childhood and society.* New York, London: W.W. Norton & Company.

Erikson, E. (1968). *Identity: Youth and crisis.* New York, London: W.W. Norton & Company.

Epping, J.E. & Willmuth, M.E. (1994). Art therapy in the rehabilitation of adolescents with spinal cord injuries: A case study. *American Journal of Art Therapy, 32,* 79–82.

Farrell Fenton, J. (2000). Cystic fibrosis and art therapy. *The Arts in Psychotherapy, 27*(1), 15–25.

Favara-Scacco, C. et al. (2001). Art therapy as support for children with leukemia during painful procedures. *Medical and Pediatric Oncology, 36,* 474–480.

Freud, A. (1958). Adolescence. *The Psychoanalytic Study of the Child, 13,* 255–278.
Freud, A. & Bergmann, T. (1965/1972). *Kranke Kinder: Ein Psychoanalytischer Beitrag zu Ihrem Verstaendnis (Engl. Original Title: Children in the hospital).* Frankfurt a.M., Germany: Fischer Verlag.
Gabriels, R.K. (1988). Art therapy assessment of coping styles in severe asthmatics. *Art Therapy,* 59–68.
Golombek, H. et al. (1989). Adolescents personality development: Three phases, three courses and varying turmoil. Findings from the Toronto Adolescent Longitudinal Study. *Canadian Journal of Psychiatry, 13,* 500–504.
Golombek, H. & Kutcher, S. (1990). Feeling states during adolescence. *Psychiatric Clinics of North America, 13,* 443–454.
Golombek, H. & Korenblum, M. (1996). Brief psychoanalytic psychotherapy with adolescents. *Adolescent Psychiatry,* 307–324.
Guenter, M. (2000). Art therapy as an intervention to stabilize the defences of children undergoing bone marrow transplantation. *The Arts in Psychotherapy, 27*(1), 3–14.
Hays, R.E. (1981). The bridge drawing: A projective technique for assessment in art therapy. *The Arts in Psychotherapy, 8,* 207–217.
Hinds, P.S. (1988). Adolescent hopefulness in illness and health. *Advances in Nursing Science, 10,* 79–88.
Hofmann, A.D. (1997). Adolescent psychosocial development. In A. Hofmann, D. & Greydanus (Eds.), *Adolescent Medicine,* 18–21. Stamford, CT: Appleton & Lange.
Hofmann, A.D. (1997). Chonic illness and hospitalization. In A. Hofmann & D. Greydanus (Eds.) *Adolescent Medicine,* 740–754. Stamford, Connecticut: Appleton & Lange.
Jaffe, Ch. M. (1991). Psychology: Psychoanalytic approaches to adolescent development. In M. Slomowitz (Ed.), *Adolescent Psychotherapy,* 13–40. Washington, DC: American Psychiatric Press, Inc.
Kimmel, P.L. (2001). Psychosocial factors in dialysis patients. *Kidney International 59,* 1599–1613.
Korenblum, M. (1998). Guidelines for the practice of psychotherapy with children and adolescents. In P. Cameron, J. Ennis, J. Peadman (Eds.) *Standards and guidelines for the psychotherapies.* Toronto: University of Toronto Press.
Kosmach, B., Corbo-Richert, B. & Pike, N. (2000). Organ transplantation. In P. Ludder Jackson & J.A. Vessey (Eds.), *Primary care of the child with a chronic condition,* 676–705. Toronto: Mosby.
Kuebler-Ross, E. (1969). *On death and dying.* New York, NY: Touchstone.
Landgarten, H.B. (1981). Rehabilitation and treatment of chronic pain. In H.B. Landgarten (Ed.), *Clinical Art Therapy,* 335–338. New York: Brunner/Mazel Publishers.
Leonhard, M.D., Rothberg, M.R. & Seiden, D. (1984). Art work of cystic fibrosis patients. *Art Therapy,* 68–74.
Linesch Greenspoon, D. (1988). *Adolescent art therapy.* New York: Brunner/Mazel Publishers.
Mackinnon, R.A. & Michels, R. (1987). *The psychiatric interview in clinical practice.* London, UK: W.B. Sanders.

Malchiodi, C.A. (1998). *The art therapy soucebook.* Los Angeles: Lowell House.
Malchiodi, C.A. (1999). *Medical art therapy with adults.* London, Philadelphia: Jessica Kingsley Publishers.
Malchiodi, C.A. (1999). *Medical art therapy with children.* London, Philadelphia: Jessica Kingsley Publishers.
Malchiodi, C.A. (2003). *Handbook of art therapy.* New York, London: The Guilford Press.
Meijer, S.A., et al. (2000). Peer interaction in adolescents with a chronic illness. *Personal and Individual Differences, 29,* 799–813.
Meijer, S.A., et al. (2002). Coping styles and locus of control as predictors for psychological adjustment of adolescents with a chronic illness. *Social Science and Medicine, 54,* 1453–1461.
Melano Flanagan, L. (1996). Object Relations Theory. In J. Berzoff, L.M. Flanagan & P. Hertz (Eds.) *Inside out and Outside in,* 127–171. Northvale NJ: Jason Aronson Inc.
Moon, B.L. (1998). *The dynamics of art as therapy with adolescents.* Springfield, IL: Charles C Thomas, Publisher, Ltd.
Moos, R.H. & Schaefer, J.A. (1984). The crisis of physical illness: An overview and conceptual analysis. In R.H. Moos (Ed.), *Coping with physical illness 2: New perspectives,* 3–25, New York: Plenum.
Musial, E.M. (1984). An unsung hero: The living related kidney donor. In R.H. Moos (Ed.), *Coping with physical illness 2: New perspectives,* 295–303, New York: Plenum.
Naumburg, M. (1966/1987). *Dynamically oriented art therapy: Its principles and practice.* Chicago: Magnolia Street Publishers.
Neinstein, L. (1991). Psychosocial development in normal adolescents. In L. Neinstein (Ed.), *Adolescent health care: A practical guide,* 39–44. Baltimore, Urban & Schwartzenberg.
Neinstein, L. (1991). Chronic physical illness in the adolescent. In L. Neinstein (Ed.), *Adolescent health care: A practical guide,* 985–1004. Baltimore, Urban & Schwartzenberg.
Oppenheim, C.C., Juszczak, L. & Wallace, N. (1984). Using creative arts to help children cope with Altered Body Image. *Child Health Care, 12*(3), 108–112.
Oster, G.D. & Gould, P. (1987). *Using drawings in assessment and therapy.* Levittown, PA: Brunner/Mazel.
Palmer, S.E., Canzona, L. & Wai L. (1984) Helping families respond effectively to chronic illness: Home dialysis as a case example. In R.H. Moos (Ed.), *Coping with physical illness 2: New perspectives,* 283–294. New York: Plenum.
Prager, A. (1993). The art therapist's role in working with hospitalized children. *American Journal of Art Therapy, 32,* 2–11.
Raghuraman, R.S. (2000). Dungeons and dragons: Dealing with emotional and behavioral issues of an adolescent with diabetes. *The Arts in Psychotherapy, 27*(1), 27–39.
Riley, S. (2001). Art therapy with adolescents. *Western Journal of Medicine, 175,* 54–57.
Riley, S. (1999). *Contemporary art therapy with adolescents.* London and Philadelphia: Jessica Kingsley, Publishers.

Rubin, J.A. (1987). *Approaches to art therapy: Theory and technique.* Bristol, PA: Brunner/Mazel.

Schultz, A.W. & Liptak, G.S. (1998). Helping adolescents who have disabilities negotiate transitions to adulthood. *Issues in Comprehensive Pediatric Nursing, 21,* 187–201.

Sacks, O. (1990). *Awakenings.* New York: Harper Perennial.

Seiffge-Krenke, I. (1998). Chronic disease and perceived developmental progression in adolescence. *Developmental Psychology, 34*(5), 1073–1084.

Silver, E.J., et al. (1990). Ego development and chronic illness in adolescents. *Journal of Personality and Social Psychology, 59*(2), 305–310.

Stapleton, S. (1983/2000). Powerlessness in persons with end-stage renal disease. In J. Fitzgerald Miller (Ed.), *Coping with chronic illness: Overcoming powerlessness,* 215–245. Philadelphia: F.A. Davis Company.

St. Clair, M. (2000). *Object relations and self psychology: An introduction.* Belmont, CA: Wadsworth/Thomson Learning.

Suris, J.C., Parera, N. & Puig, C. (1996). Chronic illness and emotional distress in adolescence. *Journal of Adolescent Health, 19,* 153–156.

Taylor, J.H. (2000). Renal failure, chronic. In P. Ludder Jackson & J.A. Vessey (Eds.), *Primary care of the child with a chronic condition,* 777–807. Toronto: Mosby.

Wadeson, H. (1980). *Art psychotherapy.* New York: John Wiley & Sons, Inc.

Wadeson, H. (1987/1995). *The dynamics of art psychotherapy.* New York: John Wiley & Sons, Inc.

Wadeson, H. (2000). Physically ill and dying children. In H. Wadeson (Ed.), *Art therapy practice,* 122–144. New York: John Willey & Sons, Inc.

Weekes, D.P. (1995). Adolescents growing up chronically ill: A life-span developmenal view. *Family and Community Health, 17*(4), 22–43.

Weldt, C. (2003). Patient's responses to a drawing experience in a hemodialysis unit: A step towards healing. *Art Therapy: Journal of the American Art Therapy Association,* 92–99.

Westhoff, K. (2001). *Bilderwelt Krebskranker Kinder.* Stuttgart, New York: Schattauer.

Winnicott, D.W. (1971/1999). Creativity and its origins. In D.W. Winnicott (Ed.), *Playing and reality,* 65–85. London, New York: Routledge.

INDEX

A

abandonment, 29, 33, 35, 179
adjunctive treatment, 27, 32
art as therapy, 23
art psychotherapy, 23
attachment, 8, 10, 24, 190
autonomy, 4, 5, 13, 14, 33
auxiliary ego, 137
avoidance, 15, 36, 180

B

bodily integrity, 34, 36, 37, 188
body image, 7, 11, 14, 21, 34, 35, 37, 179
boundary issues, 4

C

chronic renal failure, 17
client-centered therapy, 23, 41
compensation, 16
compliance, 13, 14
containment, 31
control, 4, 5, 10, 15, 23, 29, 33, 34, 177, 178
coping strategies, 15, 35, 177
countertransference, 26

D

defense mechanism, 16, 31, 37
denial, 12, 14, 16, 37, 188
dependence, 9, 10, 13, 14, 16, 21, 32, 177
disability, 13, 34, 177
displacement, 16, 31

E

early adolescence, 6, 7, 11, 12
ego strength, 3
emotion-focused control, 15, 16
end-stage renal failure, 17, 39, 177
Erikson Erik, 3, 4, 5, 6, 7, 8, 183

F

false self, 10, 190

G

good enough mother, 9, 190
grandiosity, 30

H

handicap, 13
hemodialysis, 18, 20, 41, 178, 198
holding environment, 9

I

imagining, 31, 32
immersion, 30, 32
immortality, 30
independence, 4, 9, 12, 13, 14, 20, 30, 34, 183
insight-oriented therapy, 23, 41
intellectualization, 16
internalization, 9, 32
invulnerability, 12, 30
isolation, 8, 12, 14, 21, 31, 33, 37

L

late adolescence, 6, 8, 12, 15

M

maneuvers of resistance, 30
metaphor, 29, 34
metaverbal, 28
middle adolescence, 7, 12
mistrust, 4, 7

N

narcissism, 29, 31
non-compliance, 15

O

Object Relations Theory, 8, 9, 10
objectification, 24
omnipotence, 12, 30

P

peer acceptance, 14, 29
peritoneal dialysis, 13, 18
physical integrity, 14
Pica disease, 101
post-traumatic stress disorder, 27, 36
primary control, 15
problem-focused control, 15
projection, 16
projective identification, 99
psycho-education, 35
Psychosocial Ego Development, 8
pubescence, 6

R

regression, 14, 16, 20, 31
resilience, 35, 36
resistance, 30, 31, 32, 177
reversal of affect, 31

S

secondary control, 15
secondary gain, 17
secure base, 122, 139, 148
self, 5, 6, 7, 9, 10, 22, 24, 26, 29, 33, 34, 37
self-confidence, 5, 7, 12, 34
self-esteem, 5, 7, 10, 12, 14, 23, 34, 37
self-harm, 30
sexual identity, 14
somatization, 99
stressor, 11, 15, 21, 177
suicidal ideation, 30

T

termination, 32
transference, 26
transitional object, 9
transplantation, 19, 21
true self, 10, 190

W

working alliance, 10

Y

youth, 6

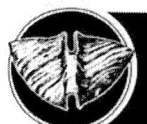

Charles C Thomas • PUBLISHER • LTD.

P.O. Box 19265
Springfield, IL 62794-9265

Complete catalog available at www.ccthomas.com

COMING SOON!

• Moon, Bruce L.—**EXISTENTIAL ART THERAPY: The Canvas Mirror** (3rd Ed.), '09, 288 pp. (7 x 10), 51 il.

• Horovitz, Ellen G. & Sarah L. Eksten—**THE ART THERAPISTS' PRIMER: A Clinical Guide to Writing Assessments, Diagnosis, and Treatment**, '09, 272 pp. (7 x 10), 106 il., 2 Tables.

NOW AVAILABLE!

• Brooke, Stephanie L.—**THE USE OF THE CREATIVE THERAPIES WITH SURVIVORS OF DOMESTIC VIOLENCE**, '08, 370 pp. (7 x 10), 57 il., (14 in color), $85.95, hard, $65.95, paper.

• Junge, Maxine Borowsky—**MOURNING, MEMORY AND LIFE ITSELF: Essays by an Art Therapist**, '08, 292 pp. (7 x 10), 38 il, $61.95, hard, $41.95, paper.

• Brooke, Stephanie L.—**THE CREATIVE THERAPIES AND EATING DISORDERS**, '08, 304 pp. (7 x 10), 20 il., 2 tables, $64.95, hard, $44.95, paper.

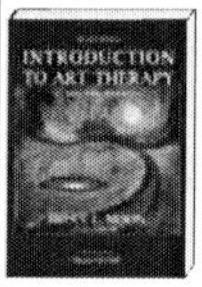

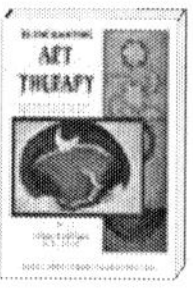

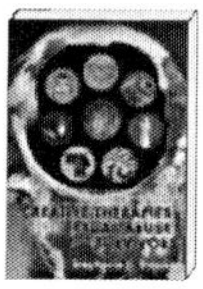

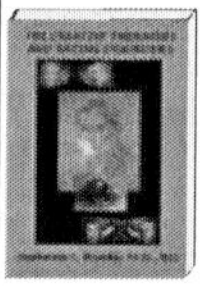

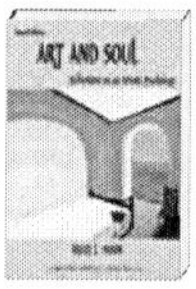

• Moon, Bruce L.—**INTRODUCTION TO ART THERAPY: Faith in the Product**, (2nd Ed.) '08, 226 pp. (7 x 10), 20 il., $53.95, hard, $33.95, paper.

• Arrington, Doris Banowsky—**ART, ANGST, AND TRAUMA: Right Brain Interventions with Developmental Issues**, '07, 278 pp. (7 x 10), 123 il. (10 in color, paper edition only), $63.95, hard, $48.95, paper.

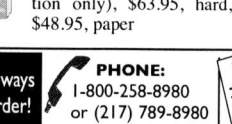

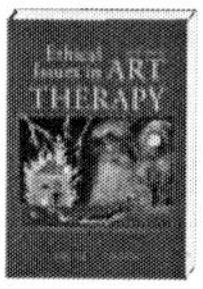

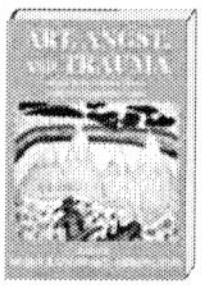

PHONE:
1-800-258-8980
or (217) 789-8980

FAX:
(217) 789-9130

EMAIL:
books@ccthomas.com

Web: www.ccthomas.com

MAIL:
Charles C Thomas
Publisher, Ltd.
P.O. Box 19265
Springfield, IL 62794-9265

5 easy ways to order!

ORDER NOW!
(see below for details on how to order)

• Moon, Bruce L.—**ETHICAL ISSUES IN ART THERAPY**, (2nd Ed.) '06, 290 pp. (7 x 10), 21 il., $56.95, hard, $38.95, paper.

• Junge, Maxine Borowsky & Harriet Wadeson—**ARCHITECTS OF ART THERAPY: Memoirs and Life Stories**, '06, 430 pp. (7 x 10), 100 il., $78.95, hard, $56.95, paper.

• Brooke, Stephanie L.—**THE USE OF THE CREATIVE THERAPIES WITH SEXUAL ABUSE SURVIVORS**, '06, 342 pp. (7 x 10), 27 il., 2 tables, $74.95, hard, $49.95, paper.

• Brooke, Stephanie L.—**CREATIVE ARTS THERAPIES MANUAL: A Guide to the History, Theoretical Approaches, Assessment, and Work with Special Populations of Art, Play, Dance, Music, Drama, and Poetry Therapies**, '06, 296 pp. (8 x 10), 34 il., 9 tables, $66.95, hard, $46.95, paper.

• Moon, Bruce L.—**ART AND SOUL: Reflections on an Artistic Psychology**, (2nd Ed.) '04, 184 pp. (6 x 9), 15 il., $44.95, hard, $28.95, paper.

• Kaplan, Lynn—**RE-ENCHANTING ART THERAPY: Transformational Practices for Restoring Creative Vitality**, '03, 304 pp. (7 x 10), 71 il., $57.95, hard, $39.95, paper.

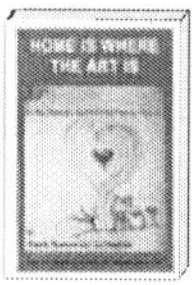

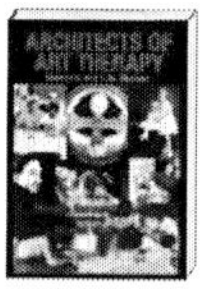

• Arrington, Doris Banowsky—**HOME IS WHERE THE ART IS: An Art Therapy Approach to Family Therapy**, '01, 294 pp. (7 x 10), 109 il. (1 in color), 18 tables, $68.95, hard, $47.95, paper.

Complete catalog available at www.ccthomas.com

• Stack, Pamela J.—**ART THERAPY ACTIVITIES: A Practical Guide for Teachers, Therapists and Parents**, '06, 154 pp. (8 1/2 x 11), $31.95, (spiral) paper.

• Stack, Pamela J.—**MY RECOVERY ZONE: An Expressive Journal for Myself**, '06, 56 pp. (8 1/2 x 11), (2 in color), $15.95, spiral (paper).

• Le Navenec, Carole-Lynne & Laurel Bridges—**CREATING CONNECTIONS BETWEEN NURSING CARE AND THE CREATIVE ARTS THERAPIES: Expanding the Concept of Holistic Care**, '05, 404 pp. (7 x 10), 33 il., 8 tables, $73.95, hard, $53.95, paper.

• Brooke, Stephanie L.—**CREATIVE ARTS THERAPIES TREATMENT: Transatlantic Dialogue**, '07, 268 pp. (7 x 10), 39 il., 1 table, $55.95, hard, $37.95, paper.

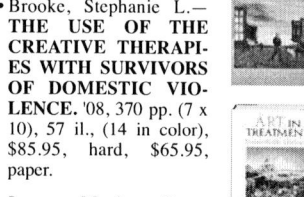

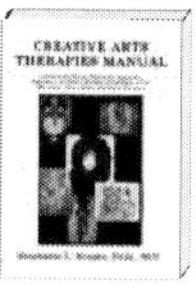

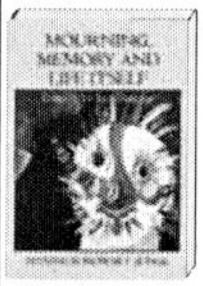

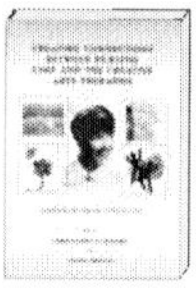

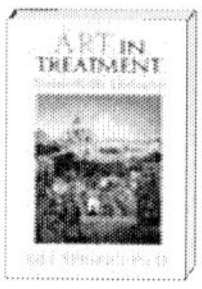

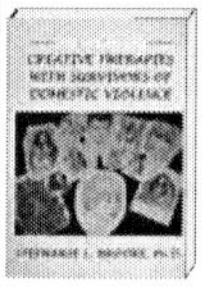

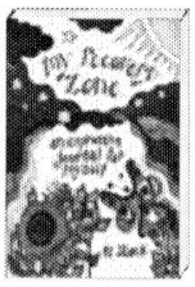

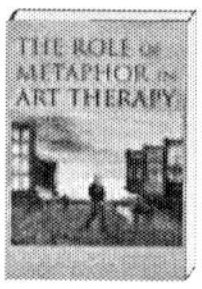

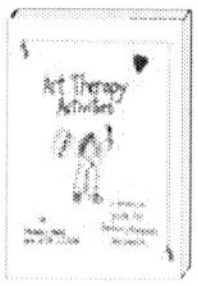

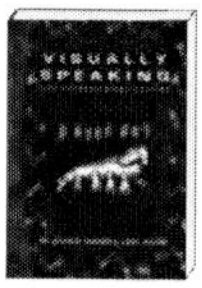

• Spring, Dee—**ART IN TREATMENT: Metaphoric Dialogue**, '07, 154 pp. (7 x 10), 16 il., $49.95, hard, $29.95, paper.

• Moon, Bruce L.—**THE ROLE OF METAPHOR IN ART THERAPY: Theory, Method, and Experience**, '07, 154 pp. (7 x 10), 16 il., $49.95, hard, $29.95, paper.

• Horovitz, Ellen G.—**VISUALLY SPEAKING: Art Therapy and the Deaf**, '07, 250 pp. (7 x 10), 71 il., 5 tables, $56.95, hard, $36.95, paper.

Books sent on approval • Shipping charges: $7.75 min. U.S. / Outside U.S., actual shipping fees will be charged • Prices subject to change without notice

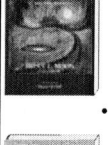

Complete catalog available at www.ccthomas.com or email books@ccthomas.com